T0140970

Pablo Mendoza Ponce

Implantable Medical Systems for the Invasive Monitoring of Pressure and Temperature

Logos Verlag Berlin

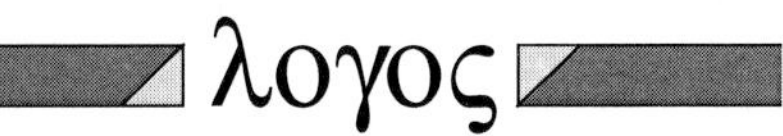

Bibliografische Information der Deutschen Nationalbibliothek

Die Deutsche Nationalbibliothek verzeichnet diese Publikation in der Deutschen Nationalbibliografie; detaillierte bibliografische Daten sind im Internet über http://dnb.d-nb.de abrufbar.

ISBN 978-3-8325-5390-6

Logos Verlag Berlin GmbH
Georg-Knorr-Str. 4, Geb. 10,
D-12681 Berlin
Germany

Tel.: +49 (0)30 / 42 85 10 90
Fax: +49 (0)30 / 42 85 10 92
http://www.logos-verlag.de

Implantable Medical Systems for the Invasive Monitoring of Pressure and Temperature

Von Promotionsausschuss der
Technischen Universität Hamburg

zur Erlangung des akademischen Grades

Doktor-Ingenieur (Dr.-Ing.)

genehmigte Dissertation

von

Pablo Mendoza Ponce

aus

San José, Costa Rica

2021

1. Gutachter: Prof. Dr.-Ing. Wolfgang H. Krautschneider
2. Gutachter: Prof. Dr.-Ing. Alexander Schlaefer

Tag der mündlichen Prüfung: 26. August 2021

To my beloved parents Antonio and Ana.

To my dear Anna and Benjamin.

Abstract

This dissertation presents research on the design and implementation of structures for a miniaturised implantable medical system (IMS) to continuously monitor the interstitial fluid pressure and temperature in the body of animals or humans. The information from these variables is vital for physicians and researchers. For instance, cancer research has found a relationship between these bio-parameters and the evolution of a microenvironment that intensifies a tumour's growth behaviour. In the area of pressure measurement, two alternatives for a miniaturised IMS are evaluated: piezoresistive and capacitive pressure transducers. For both types of transducers, a noise analysis is used to define the requirements and design parameters for their interfaces. Furthermore, to verify the performance of the proposed designs, prototypes of such interfaces were implemented and fabricated as part of test chips. Regarding the tumour temperature monitoring, the design and implementation results of an on-chip temperature transducer unit are presented. Moreover, to run these devices, a low-power timing and clock generation unit was developed and implemented. An IMS prototype for the continuous monitoring of pressure and temperature was designed and fabricated. The encapsulation process and mechanical details of such a system are described. The IMS prototype was tested using human cancer xenografts grown in SCID mice without any therapeutic applied. A calibration sequence for the prototype system sensing units is described. The devices were able to run autonomously for 48 hours after every charge cycle. The recorded data showed increasing pressure and decreasing temperature in the tumour following the implantation, which is consistent with the findings from other research groups that have studied growing tumours.

Acknowledgements

It is my pleasure to express my gratefulness to all those who helped me from day zero to put all these ideas together into something concrete that one day might help humanity. I would like to express my special thanks to the heads of the Institute for Integrated Circuits (formerly Institute for Medial Electronics) Prof. Dr.-ing. Wolfgang Krautschneider and Prof. Dr-ing. Matthias Kuhl, who gave me the precious opportunity to work in this academic department, and which also guided me through the path of a researcher. I am profoundly thankful to them.

As I have found throughout my professional career, a research project success also depends on all those colleagues around you, and this project is no exception. I am indebted to my colleagues and friends in the Hamburg University of Technology, specially to Dr. Ing. Lait Abu-Saleh, Gayas M. Sayed, Johan Solis Arbustini, Dr.-Ing. habil. Dietmar Schröder, Dr. Ing. Rajeev Ranjan and Dr. Ing. Bibin John. As well, the staff at the institute, Ute, Ronald, Gaby, and Silke. To them and many others that influenced my work in the last few years, I will always be grateful.

I wish to acknowledge the constant support and love from my family, my wife, Anna; my son, Benji (also for being patient); my mother, Ana; my brothers, Pedro and Moisés; as well as my extended family, Kem, Joyce, Terry, Sarah and Edie. Not less important, for the supporting words of close friends around the world, Catterina, Nishma, Diego, Dora, Victor, David M, David L, Sebas, Marta V., Migue, Maria, Lizeth, Lidieth and Monica. Many thanks from my hearth.

Finally, I truly appreciated the economical and technical contribution from the Instituto Tecnológico de Costa Rica, TUHH, Institute for Integrated Circuits, Institut für Flugzeug-Systemtechnik, FMTHH and UKE. Without their support and funding, this project could not have been successful.

Contents

List of Figures

List of Tables

List of Abbreviations

ΣΔM	Sigma-Delta Modulator
ADC	Analogue-to-Digital Converter
AFE	Analogue front-end
AIMD	Active Implantable Medical Device Directive
ASIC	Application-Specific Integrated Circuit
BJT	Bipolar Junction Transistors
CCO	current controlled oscillator
CDC	Capacitance-to-Digital Converter
CMOS	Complementary Metal Oxide Semiconductor
CSV	Comma Separated Values
CTAT	Complementary to absolute temperature
CTC	Capacitance-to-Time Converter
CVC	Capacitance-to-Voltage Converter
ECM	Extracellular Matrix
ENOB	Effective Number of Bits
FPGA	Field-Programmable Gate Array
HIF-1 α	Hypoxia-inducible factor–1α
IΣΔADC	Incremental Sigma-Delta ADC
IFP	Interstitial Fluid Pressure
IMS	Implantable Medical System
INL	Integral Non Linearity error
LDO	Low Dropout

LSB	Least Significative Bit
MEMS	Microelectromechanical Systems
N-MOS	N-type Metal-Oxide Semiconductor
OSR	Oversampling Ratio
OTA	Operational Transconductance Amplifier
P-MOS	P-type Metal-Oxide Semiconductor
PCB	Printed Circuit Board
PoR	Power-on-Reset
PSD	Power Spectral Density
PTFE	Polytetrafluoroethylene
PVT	Process, Supply Voltage, and Temperature
QFN	Quad Flat No-leads
RMS	root mean square
SAR	Succesive-Approximation Register
SCID	Severe Combined Immunodeficiency
SPI	Serial Peripheral Interface
TDC	Time-to-Digital Converter
TGF-β	Transforming Growth Factor Beta
VEGF	Vascular Endothelial Growth Factor
VTC	Voltage-to-Time Converter

Physical Constants

Boltzmann constant	$k_B = 1.380\,649 \times 10^{-23}\,\mathrm{J\,K^{-1}}$
Electron charge	$q = 1.602\,176\,62 \times 10^{-19}\,\mathrm{C}$
Vacuum dielectric constant	$\epsilon_0 = 8.854\,19 \times 10^{-12}\,\mathrm{F\,m^{-1}}$
Silicon band-gap energy	$E_g = 1.11\,\mathrm{eV}$ @ $300\,\mathrm{K}$

List of Symbols

A_{AFE}	Analogue front-end gain.	-
B_{AFE}	Analogue front-end frequency bandwidth.	Hz
B_{bridge}	Piezoresistive sensor frequency bandwidth.	Hz
$C_{\mathrm{in,AFE}}$	Analogue front-end input capacitance.	F
C_{offset}	Capacitive sensor offset capacitance.	F
C_{par}	Parasitic capacitance.	F
C_{sens}	Capacitive sensor nominal capacitance.	F
E	Young modulus.	Pa
$i_{\mathrm{n,dis}}$	Noise component from the current reference circuit (CTC).	A
J_{L}	Lymphatic drainage flux.	$\mathrm{m^3\,s^{-1}}$
J_{s}	Net fluid flux between capillary and interstitial space.	$\mathrm{m^3\,s^{-1}}$
L_{m}	Hydraulic conductivity of the membrane.	$\mathrm{m^2\,s\,kg^{-1}}$
$N_{\mathrm{o,ADC}}$	Total noise produced in the ADC.	$\mathrm{V^2}$
$N_{\mathrm{o,AFE}}$	Total noise produced in the analogue front-end.	$\mathrm{V^2}$
$N_{\mathrm{o,bridge}}$	Total noise produced in a piezoresistive transducer.	$\mathrm{V^2}$
$N_{\mathrm{o,sys}}$	Total noise in the data path for the piezoresistive sensor.	$\mathrm{V^2}$

p_{r}	Pressure resolution.	mmHg
p_{c}	Hydrostatic pressure in the capillary.	mmHg
p_{isf}	Hydrostatic pressure of the interstitial fluid.	mmHg
R_{pzr}	Piezoresistive element electrical resistance.	Ω
S_{pzr}	Piezoresistive transducer sensitivity.	mV/VmmHg
T	Temperature.	K
T_{clk}	Period of the clock generation unit output signal.	s
t_{d}, t_{dc}	CMOS thyristor time delay.	s
$t_{\mathrm{n,ctc-1}}$	Total time uncertainty added by the differential thyristor pair (CTC).	s
$t_{\mathrm{n,ctc-2}}$	Total time uncertainty added by the pulse generator (CTC).	s
$t_{\mathrm{n,i,d}x}$	Time uncertainty added during the discharging phase of capacitor x (CTC).	s
$t_{\mathrm{n,osc}}$	Jitter introduced by the relaxation oscillator (TDC).	s
$t_{\mathrm{n,v,c}x}$	Time uncertainty added during the charging phase of capacitor x (CTC).	s
$T_{\mathrm{osc-timer}}$	Period of the timer output signal.	s
$t_{V\mathrm{out-ref}}$	Time delay generated by the reference capacitance thyristor branch (at the CTC).	s
$t_{V\mathrm{out-sens}}$	Time delay generated by the capacitive transducer thyristor branch (at the CTC).	s
V_{bridge}	Output voltage of a Wheatstone bridge.	V
$V_{\mathrm{dd,bridge}}$	Piezoresistive transducer supply voltage.	V
V_{EB}	Emitter-base voltage of a BJT transistor	V
$V_{\mathrm{EB,d}}$	Emitter-base voltage of a Darlington configuration.	V
V_{H}	Hooge noise in a piezoresistive sensor.	V
V_{J}	Johnson noise in a piezoresistive sensor.	V
V_{jitter}	Phase noise (due to jitter in the sampling block of an ADC).	V

$v_{\text{ktc}x,\text{tc}}$	kTC Noise introduced at the end of the charging phase of capacitor x in the (CTC).	V
$v_{\text{n,c}x}$	Total output voltage uncertainty at capacitor x (sense or reference) in the CTC.	V
$v_{\text{n,vdd,tc}}$	Noise introduced by the voltage supply at the end of the charging phase of capacitor x in the CTC.	V
$v_{\text{o,AFE}}$	Noise at the output of the piezoresistive analogue front-end.	V
$v_{\text{o,bridge}}$	Noise at the output of a piezoresistive sensor.	V
$V_{\text{quantisation}}$	Quantisation noise in an ADC.	V
V_{thermal}	Thermal noise in an ADC.	V
V_{thp}	PMOS transistor threshold voltage.	V
V_{thn}	NMOS transistor threshold voltage.	V
V_{TM}	Thermomechanical noise in a piezoresistive sensor.	V
W_{ADC}	Weight for the ADC bridge noise contribution.	-
W_{AFE}	Weight for the analogue front-end bridge noise contribution.	-
W_{bridge}	Weight for the piezoresistive bridge noise contribution.	-
Δt_{CTC}	Capacitance to time converter output time difference.	s
γ_{s}	Strain.	-
ν	Poisson's ratio.	-
π_{c}	Colloid pressure in the capillary.	mmHg
π_{isf}	Colloid pressure in the interstitial fluid.	mmHg
ρ	Electrical resistivity.	$\Omega\,\text{m}$
σ_{ov}	Osmotic reflection coefficient of the vessel wall.	-
σ_{qCDC}	Quantisation noise introduced by the TDC.	s

Chapter 1

Introduction

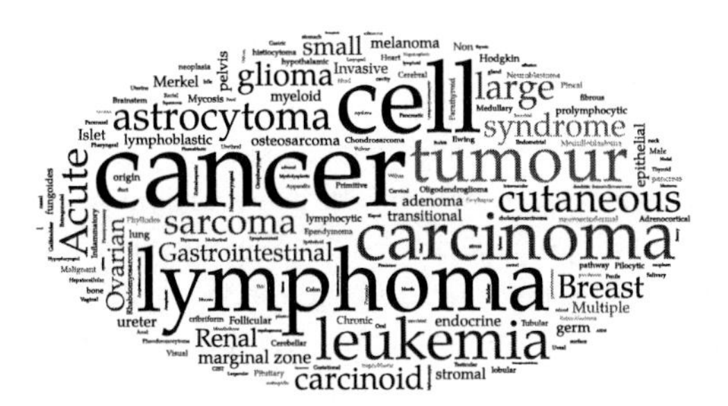

The generations born after the Second World War (mainly in developed countries) have benefited from the cradle to the grave welfare thanks to innovations in medicine as well as a relatively stable economic and social environment. Moreover, and due to these life improvements, nowadays, a significant proportion of the human population has high chances to live into or even beyond their sixties, a positive figure; however, an ageing population also means more people requiring quality healthcare. Therefore, today is the time to innovate and improve medicine through technology, so that the future continuous looking bright.

With the increase in population, and especially an ageing one, certain diseases have become prevalent, and cancer is one of them. In 2018, different types of cancer affected around 18.1 million persons. Furthermore, 9.6 million lives were lost to cancer, representing a third of all premature deaths from non-communicable diseases in adults [1]. However, in the past decades, medical research has not only worked on finding new treatments but to also unveiling the mechanisms that help a tumour to grow and develop. Henceforth, it is prevailing to use each new finding on cancer to produce better technology to help in the cause to cure cancer.

Computer Tomography (CT) and Magnetic Resonance Imaging (MRI) are two of the most used standard techniques for screening, diagnosing and evaluating tumours [2]. These techniques are complementary, and the use of one or the other depends on the type of cancer. However, their use is not always possible due to health risks. CT has a radiation risk involved, and therefore a patient can only undergo a limited number of exams. MRI, and also CT, might require the use of a contrast dye which could trigger allergic reactions. Additionally, the availability of MRI and CT devices in the health systems is by far not large enough for getting the necessary number of exams for continuous monitoring (e.g., in 2013, the average number of MRI and CT units per hundred thousand people in the European Union countries was 1.21 and 1.86, respectively [3, 4]).

As described, the predominant imaging methods (e.g., CT and MRI) for diagnosing and evaluating cancer provide a limited number of samples over time. Furthermore, these limitations result in a significant loss of physiological information that has the potential to bring physicians and researchers a better understanding of the disease evolution. Conversely, miniaturised, semi-autonomous implantable monitoring systems for the continuous measurement of biophysical, biochemical and metabolic variables provides a solution to the limitations described. Therefore, the design of an implantable system for the continuous monitoring of tumours would help to improve current therapies and might help researchers to get a new tool to study cancer.

The conjunction between electronics and medicine has transformed medical research and health care in the last century. Even more, in the last decades, the accelerated development in technologies such as microelectronics and microfabrication has opened tremendous opportunities to develop smaller yet more sophisticated medical electronic systems. This wave of innovation opens the door to new opportunities to develop new or improve therapy and diagnosis tools. Therefore, and given the need for tools to fight cancer, the development of miniaturised implantable systems is an exciting field in the electronics research area.

1.1 Purpose of the work

The use of an implantable system for cancer monitoring provides several advantages, from which the most important is the possibility of continuous monitoring of the tumour physiological variables. In the present work, the main goal is to set the foundations for the development of a miniaturised implantable monitoring system for the continuous evaluation of the pressure and temperature in tumours. In this way, this document aims to provide the theoretical background regarding the development of the sensing units and the sampling control used in such implantable system. Furthermore, a set of in-vivo experiments were designed to verify the implantable system concept using a prototype unit.

During the development of this work, to achieve the goal previously described the focus was set on the following tasks:

- Define, analyse and implement options for the monitoring of pressure and temperature in a tumour.
- Design and implement a low-power timing unit for low-data rate implantable systems.
- Investigate and test alternatives for the encapsulation (to protect both the implantable system and the host) of an implantable system.
- Produce a prototype implantable system for the measurement of pressure and temperature in tumour xenografts.
- Perform in-vivo experiments with the prototype to prove the implantable system concept.

The final result of this work is the proof-of-concept experiments. These experiments were performed in cooperation with the Universitaẗsklinikum Hamburg-Eppendorf. With these experiments, it was intended to verify the measuring interfaces developed in a real scenario. Figure 1.1 presents the

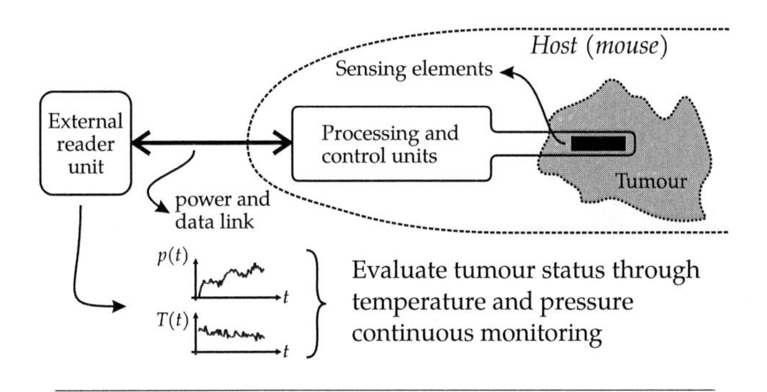

FIGURE 1.1: Basic concept of the developed system.

concept for the proof-of-concept experiments. The prototype system holds the temperature and pressure sensors, interfaces, control circuitry and power storage units. During the experiments, the sensing units in the implantable system prototype are placed inside a tumour xenograft (grown inside a mouse). An external unit is used to provide charge to the implantable system and to read the data gathered by it. The charge received by the implant allows it to perform several measurements autonomously for several days. Here it is relevant to highlight that this work was delimited to study the autonomous bio-parameters acquisition using an implantable system (i.e. the pressure and temperature sensing). Therefore, other blocks (e.g., the data and power link) where implemented straightforwardly and robustly, so that do not interfere with the characterisation of the units under study.

This work has been partially supported by a grant from Tecnoloǵico de Costa Rica with number 37-2015-D and also by the German Exist program and European Social Funding with number 03EFKHH024.

1.2 Thesis Outline

This document is structured as follows: Chapter 2 introduces the concept of implantable medical systems and its design challenges. The biological background of the interstitial space, the area of interest to measure pressure and temperature, is presented in the second part of this chapter.

Chapters 3 and 4 present the theory behind pressure and temperature monitoring, respectively. These two chapters describe the design of sensors to translate these physiological variables into an equivalent digital form. Furthermore, integrated circuit implementations and experimental results are presented for each sensor. Similarly, the design, implementation and verification of a timing unit for the implantable system are described in Chapter 5. Chapter 6 explains the considerations for encapsulation and mechanics for the implantable system prototype.

The first part of Chapter 7 explains the importance of monitoring pressure and temperature in a tumour. The second part presents the design and implementation of an implantable system prototype for the measurement of pressure and temperature in tumours. Additionally, this chapter describes the results obtained from in-vivo tests performed using the developed prototype. Finally, the summary and the future outlook of this work are presented in Chapter 8.

Chapter 2

Fundamentals

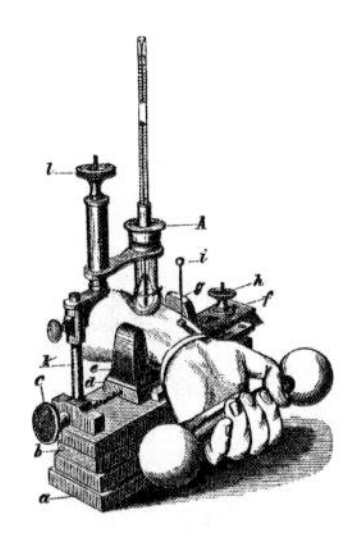

[5]

The monitoring of body parameters under traditional medicine practice is limited. Unless the patient remains in a hospital bed continuously connected to equipment, physicians only have access to a limited number of samples of these variables on each visit. This last point represents a problem to get a complete characterisation of a patient's condition. However, implantable medical systems provide a solution for better monitoring of health conditions.

In this chapter, a brief introduction to electronic medical implantable systems is provided. The challenges of encapsulation and integrated circuits design for IMS are also presented. Furthermore, the development of medical systems requires an understanding of the role played by the biological parameters under monitoring. In the case of this work, the implantable systems aim to measure the interstitial fluid pressure. Therefore in the second part of this chapter, a description and a model of the interstitial space is presented.

2.1 Implantable Medical Systems

The area of electronics dealing with the theory and methodology for the research and development of devices and instruments for healthcare is called Medical electronics. The intention behind these devices and instruments is to improve human life by providing better diagnosis and treatment for diverse diseases. Furthermore, medical research is also benefited from electronics by procuring tools to measure, monitor, and analyse biological signals and markers.

Implantable Medical System (IMS) is a subdivision of medical electronics that delve with apparatuses that are intended to function inside the body of a person or test subject (in case of research it can be human or animal). Based on their functionality, Implantable systems can be classified in one of the following categories (but not restricted to these) :

- An electro-stimulating device. These are devices that provide controlled and periodic electrical pulses to specific muscles, nerves, or regions in the brain. The goal of these pulses is to pace a diseased organ; examples of these devices are pacemakers and implants for Parkinson treatment.
- An automated drug delivery system able to apply the drug not just in a highly localised area but also in the exact time and quantity. With this, treatments become more effective, and their side effects are reduced. A commercial example is implantable insulin pumps.
- A bio-signal recording unit. Examples of these are implantable devices used for getting access to Electrocardiogram (ECG), Electromyogram (EMG), and Electroencephalogram (EEG) signals inside the body. These devices help clinicians and researchers to get better signal quality by avoiding problems related to the use of external electrodes (on the skin).
- A biological marker monitoring system. These devices are equipped with one or more sensors for reading vital parameters such as pressure, temperature, pH, among others. These units can be used to check the status of different conditions on the human body.

In the legal field, the classification of medical systems depends on several factors, as their invasiveness, the risk to the patient and operators associated with a failure of the device, among others. In the United States of America, the Food and Drug Administration (FDA) is the entity responsible for regulating medical devices and instruments. Title 21, Code of Federal Regulations (CFR), presents the basic rules about medical devices [6]. The CFR device volume, Parts 862-892, describes the classification of about 1700 device types into three classes [7]:

- **Class I**: Low health risk devices since most are used for external use. Some general controls are applied to these medical elements (e.g., registration of the product and manufacturer with the FDA and correct labelling, among others).
- **Class II**: Devices with medium health risk. General controls apply, as well as special controls regarding labelling, performance standards and monitoring of the devices post-marketing.
- **Class III**: This classification covers devices for life-support/sustaining, therefore presenting the higher risks. The added regulation layer (over the general and special rules) represents the most stringent control. The devices in this class require to pass a clinical evaluation to prove their safety and effectiveness. This in-depth scrutiny is needed to get approved for commercialisation.

In the case of the European Union (EU), a harmonised, community-wide legislation is worked by the EU commission. The directives derived from this legislation is implemented by competent authorities nominated by each member state. The competent authorities designate notified bodies which certify medical devices and verify conformity disputes with manufacturers. The directives present the requirements that medical products have to comply. The free circulation of a medical product in the European market is possible only when it complies with the directives ruling its type of device. The CE-mark demonstrates the approval of a device in all the EU and the European Free Trade Association. Three directives address the EU medical products legislation: the In Vitro Diagnostics Directive (IVD), the Medical Device Directive (MD) and the Active Implantable Medical Device Directive (AIMD); being the last one applicable for the present work [6].

The AIMD (adopted in 1990) deals with those devices that possess an energy source and are implanted in the human body (partially or entirely). The rules contained in this directive describe safety requirements, such as the need for sterility or protection against electrical hazards, among others [6].

The EU classification, as the USA (FDA) one, is based on the estimated risk a product represents to the patient or operators. In this way, the EU classifies medical devices into four categories [6]:

- **Class I:** Represents the lowest level of risk. There is no need for certification, and the device complies with the essential requirements is the sole manufacturer responsibility; however, if the product is sterile or is a measuring device, a notified body assessment is required. Typical examples are gauze, corrective glasses, and wheelchairs.

- **Class IIa:** The design of these devices is self-certified, but there is an independent verification and certification of its production. These devices are characterised to be used for short periods (less than a month). Contact lenses are examples of devices in this class.
- **Class IIb:** Products in this category present a higher risk than those in class IIa. The patient uses these devices for longer than one month. In the case of products, both design and production are certified by the notified body.
- **Class III:** This is the highest risk level; therefore, it requires monitoring during its lifetime. These devices require approval before entering the market. Specialised entities do the monitoring of these devices.

2.1.1 General Architecture

Figure 2.1 shows the general diagram of an implantable monitoring system. One or more transducers are used to sense various biological signals or markers of interest for the application. A set of interfaces is set for conditioning and digitising the electrical output from the transducers. Furthermore, in modern implementations, this path consists of not only electronic components, but also software (e.g., digital filters and compensation algorithms, among others). These software units can be either entirely implemented in the IMS or reside partially on the reader-hardware.

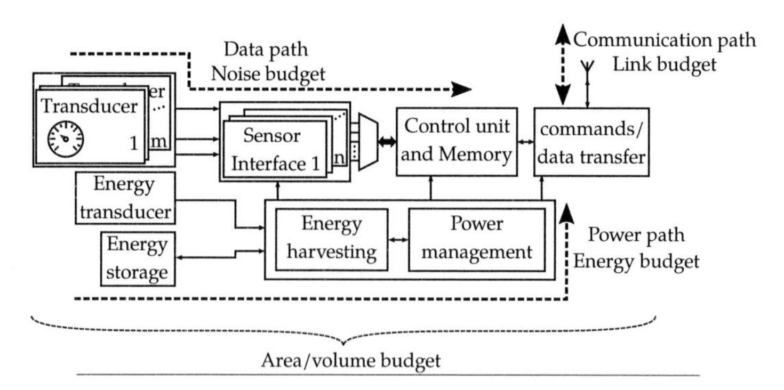

FIGURE 2.1: General block diagram of a medical implantable monitoring system.

The elements previously described conform the data-path, and a noise budget defines its specifications. The data-path is critical to provide the needed resolution for the measured quantities. The usual design flow for this part consists of first defining the accuracy and precision goals for the parameters to measure. These requirements are defined together with health experts. With these specifications, it is then possible to select the appropriate transducer elements and calculate a noise budget for the entire data-path. The noise allowed in the system provides a way to constraint the uncertainty added by the elements (hardware and software) in the path of each sensor. Each element is then designed to meet these constraints; therefore, an accurate noise model of them is required.

The power path is defined by an energy budget and consists of a set of energy elements, an optional energy harvesting unit, and a power management block. The IMS might use an energy storage element, an energy harvesting transducer, or both as power elements. For long-term IMS, energy harvesting is preferred over the use of single-use batteries to avoid the need of surgical interventions for battery replacement (or a full device replacement when the packaging does not allow access to the depleted battery). Additionally, the energy storage element can be rechargeable or not. The size of the energy storage element and the energy consumption of the system determines the level of autonomy the IMS can reach.

A communication path is set between the IMS and the external world. The characteristics (e.g. bit-rate, link distance, power required) of this path depend on the implantation depth, the type of link (e,g, inductive, RF, ultrasonic) and the external reader hardware. For a generic IMS, the communication link provides some (or all) of the following functions [8]:

- Indicate the presence of an IMS and provide information about it to authorised personnel (e.g., physicians).
- Provide access to command to activate and deactivate of the IMS on demand.
- Straightforward and secure handling of the device configuration.
- Provide a channel for fail-safe upgrade of the device firmware.
- Commands to take manual control of the IMS.

- Access to the information collected by the IMS sensing units, device parameters, and status registers, as well as commands for device diagnostics.

Of high importance for modern IMS is that the communication link provides as high information security protocols as possible. The previous is critical not only to keep the information unseen by unauthorised users but also to prevent someone from altering the IMS configuration in such a way that produces malfunction or harm to the patient carrying it.

2.1.2 Challenges for IC design

The design of integrated circuits for IMS present particular challenges when compared to the requirements for most industrial applications. However, due to the nature of the human body, specific requirements, as the operating temperature range, are less stringent (i.e., for industrial applications, a typical operating temperature is −40 °C to 85 °C, while for the body should remain around 37 °C) [7].

One of the most stringent constraints on the IC design for IMS is the power consumption. The small volume requirements for IMS limit the size of energy storage or harvesting units, meaning that the circuitry in the IMS has to function with a tiny energy budget. The most straightforward technique to reduce power consumption, without compromising the performance of the different components in the IMS is to turn off, the units that are not in use. However, some blocks as the power management or volatile memory blocks cannot be shut down, therefore need to be highly optimised for energy usage. Furthermore, as the size and threshold voltages of transistors are scaled-down in modern CMOS technologies, the leakage currents are increased, resulting in higher energy consumption even for blocks inactive [9, 10].

The Monitoring IMS makes use of a substantial amount of analogue blocks. Due to the power restrictions, a common practice is to design these blocks in the subthreshold regime. IMS designers take vantage of the relatively low speeds needed for processing biological signals and parameters (e.g., the typical sampling rate for EEG is between 250 Hz and 2000 Hz [11]). Besides, the reduced temperature variation experienced in the human body results in less restrictive considerations regarding the design temperature dependencies. However, the process variations over the threshold voltage can hurt the design [9]; therefore, special care has to be taken to reduce their impact or to compensate it.

A second challenge has to do with wireless communication and power links used by IMS. Each tissue in the human body has a certain degree of conductivity and presents different dielectric parameters. In this way, there is a high loss in the wireless links between the IMS and the external reader units. Furthermore, the radiation patterns are highly influenced by the location of the IMS in the body. The previous limits the power received by the energy harvester units in the IMS, as well as to low SNR in the communication link [10]. The first problem is solved (as previously described) by power usage optimisation. In the case of the resulting low SNR in the communication, part of it is solved with a robust front-end in the reader hardware; however, the IMS has to implement coding schemes to improve the BER, which adds complexity to the system.

Finally, the legal framework that regulates IMS can present challenges for the design of the circuits. For instance, for wireless devices, the links have to comply with the Industrial, Scientific and Medical (ISM), limiting the possibilities on frequency selection. Furthermore, standards set limits on the radiation specific absorption rate, which restricts the maximum power transmitted through the body, which results on limits on power and SNR [12].

2.1.3 Device encapsulation

Typically, the electronic components of an IMS are not biocompatible; additionally, the fluids and tissues in the human body represent a harsh environment for common electronic elements. The encapsulation of IMS into a biocompatible and hemocompatible material case solves these previously described problems. However, the device encapsulation represents a challenge for the development of IMS [13].

As mentioned, the encapsulation, which can be hard or soft, guarantees the reliability and performance of an IMS during the time is implanted (usually its lifetime). The reliability of this encasing is crucial, as any malfunction might translate into discomfort in the best case, permanent damage, even worse, death. The selection of the hardness of the encasing depends on the application, where hard encapsulations are preferred when high-stress levels are expected. In contrast, soft encapsulations allows the system to adapt to the spaces in soft-tissue. Furthermore, designers require to find a balance between the thickness of the encapsulation (directly related to the degree of protection) and the IMS size [14].

2.2 Interstitial space and its characteristics

The area in between cells, typically filled with proteins and fluid, is known as the interstitial space. The fluid filling this region has a similar composition as plasma; however, there is a difference in the protein concentration [15]. Concerning the human body, this distributed region represents about a sixth of its total volume. The interstitial space, the micro-circulatory and the lymphatic systems are essential on a large number of physiological (as well as pathological) processes. These systems regulate the exchange of oxygen, nutrients, waste products, small molecules (e.g., sugars), small plasma proteins, solutes, hormones, leukocytes, and gases as oxygen and carbon dioxide. The processes involved in these exchanges take place between the capillaries and the interstitial space [16, 17].

The gradients of pressure found in the interface between the blood capillaries and the interstitial space determine their exchange of fluids. In 1896, British physiologist Ernest Starling defined the relationship of the different forces that drive the circulation between the interstitial area and the capillary [18]. In this way, the Starling equation defines the net fluid flux J_s ($\mathrm{m^3\,s^{-1}}$) at any point in the interface between the capillary and the interstitial space as [17, 19]:

$$J_\mathrm{s} = L_\mathrm{m} A \left[p_\mathrm{c} - p_\mathrm{isf} - \sigma_\mathrm{ov}(\pi_\mathrm{c} - \pi_\mathrm{isf}) \right] , \tag{2.1}$$

where σ_ov is the osmotic reflection coefficient of the vessel wall (adimensional, 0 for a fully permeable membrane and 1 for an impermeable one), L_m and A are the hydraulic conductivity ($\mathrm{m^2\,s\,kg^{-1}}$), and the surface area ($\mathrm{m^2}$) of the blood capillary, respectively. Moreover, p_x and π_x are the hydrostatic and colloid (oncotic) pressures at the region x (sub-index isf for the interstitial area and c for the blood capillary), respectively.

For this relationship, it is essential to understand the role played by each pressure component and their behaviour on healthy tissue. The different pressure components involved in the Starling equation and a representation of the magnitude and direction of the flow along the capillary length are presented in Figure 2.2. In the case of the interstitial space, there are two pressure components involved in the fluid exchange, the negative hydrostatic pressure p_isf, whose value stays in the range −1 mmHg to −3 mmHg [16],

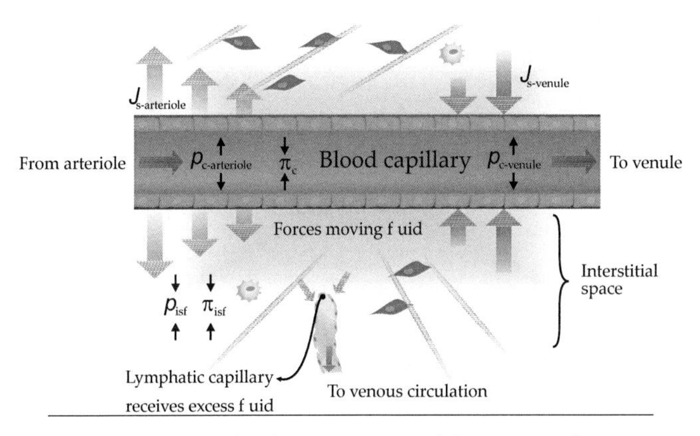

FIGURE 2.2: Graphical representation of the interstitial space and its interactions with the blood and lymphatic capillaries in normal tissue [16, 20].

and the interstitial fluid osmotic (oncotic) π_{isf} pressure (generated from the proteins and proteoglycans in this region [21]) with an average value of 8 mmHg [16]. Both pressure components in the interstitial space have a net action of pulling fluid from the capillary (represented in Figure 2.2 with arrows pointing towards the variables p_{isf} and π_{isf}).

The other two components that regulate the fluid flow (as per Equation 2.1) are related to the microcirculation characteristics in the blood capillary. The first component is the plasma oncotic pressure π_{c}, with a value of around 28 mmHg [15, 22]. As shown in Figure 2.2, this pressure component has the effect of holding the fluid within the capillary (i.e., favours fluid resorption). The second component in the blood capillary is its hydrostatic pressure p_{c}, whose effect is of pushing the fluid out of the capillary. This pressure component presents a gradient in the direction of the normal blood flow. In this way, at the arterial end, the hydrostatic capillary pressure has an average value in the range 25 mmHg to 35 mmHg, which combined (Equation 2.1) with the other three pressure components previously described results into a net flow towards the interstitial tissue.

In the case of the venous end of the capillary, the hydrostatic pressure can fall to as low as 15 mmHg [22]. Due to this reduction on the hydrostatic pressure, the net fluid flow is reversed and therefore favours the fluid resorption. In this way, there is a bidirectional exchange of biological and chemical components between the bloodstream and the tissue. Also, it is essential to note the crucial role played by the lymphatic system by taking any exceeding fluid out of the interstitial space. The effect of the lymphatic drainage J_L in the interstitial area can be added in the Starling equation so that the model becomes [18]:

$$J_\mathrm{s} = L_\mathrm{m} A \left[p_\mathrm{c} - p_\mathrm{isf} - \sigma_\mathrm{ov}(\pi_\mathrm{c} - \pi_\mathrm{isf}) \right] - J_\mathrm{L} , \tag{2.2}$$

This final relationship provides a complete picture, from the pressure point of view, of the dynamics in a healthy interstitial space. As it would be described in detail on the next chapters, the presence of a tumour affects the biological balance on its surroundings, creating a microenvironment that amplifies the tumour malignancy.

Chapter 3

Pressure Monitoring

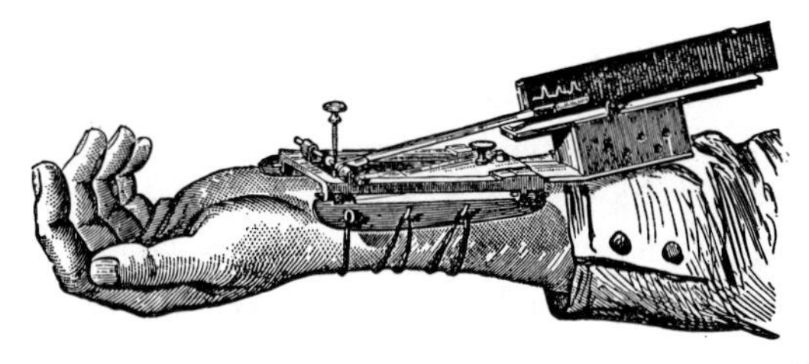

[23]

Pressure monitoring has been a vital diagnosis and study tool for physicians and researchers since the XVIII century. For instance, blood pressure studies go back to the experiments of Stephen Hales in 1733 [24]. On this first experiment, Hales inserted a short brass pipe connected to a larger vertical glass tube into a mare's crural artery and observed that

> the Blood rose in the Tube eight Feet three Inches perpendicular above the Level of the left Ventricle of the Heart; But it did not attain to its full Height at once; it rushed up about half way in an Instant, and afterwards gradually at each Pulse twelve, eight, six, four, two, and sometimes one Inch; When it was at its full Height, it would rise and fall at and after each Pulse two, three, or four Inches; ... [25, p. 1-2]

This very invasive method opened the door to research on the behaviour of pressure in the cardiovascular system. However, innovation in this field had to wait about a century for Carl Ludwig to develop the kymograph (from Greek *kuma-*, swell or wave + -graph, writing) which enabled a representation of the blood pressure to be drawn on a drum. This device was based on the use of mercury for blood pressure monitoring from Poiseuille [24]. Nevertheless, these inventions still required operation to access the internal blood pressure. It was not until 1855 that Vierordt designed his Sphygmograph (from Greek *sphygmo-*, pulse + -graph) [24]. Vierordt's Sphygmograph was based on measuring the pressure needed to obliterate the radial pulse. Etienne Jules Marey developed an improved design in 1860 (shown as this chapter art illustration), which was used mostly on research. Modern blood pressure measurement became established through on further improved designs (i.e. use of an inflatable arm cuff by Riva-Rocci in 1896) that lead to the differentiation of diastolic and systolic blood pressure [24].

Together with the discoveries and innovation in blood pressure monitoring, researchers and physicians have found that pressure plays an essential role in various bodily functions and that monitoring pressure in diverse areas of the body allows the assessment of health conditions. In light of this, the monitoring of the intracranial, intraocular, urethral, and interstitial pressure (among others) are all interesting fields of study, where innovation in sensing methods is a must. Over the history of blood pressure monitoring, each new method has sought further comfort for the patient, and increased information reliability.

Miniaturised pressure sensors have revolutionised the way physicians access this parameter. By integrating these units into micro-catheters, implantable pressure sensors became one of the first sensing micro-systems to be implantable[26]. Nowadays these small devices are found in multiple applications; from glaucoma treatment to intracranial pressure monitoring, as well as on wearable units for non-invasive e-health applications. With these devices present in more and more areas of health, it has become clear that daily readings of pressure far surpass in-clinic measurements in usefulness [27]. The development of low-power, small area and robust ways to continuously monitor pressure is therefore necessary.

This chapter presents a discussion on methods and devices for the measurement of pressure. The first part outlines the miniaturised transducers used for the translation of pressure into electrical signals. After this, the second part explains the techniques used for processing the information from the transducer and its digitisation. Furthermore, for each interface type, a noise analysis is presented.

3.1 MEMs pressure transducers

Transducers are electronic elements used to translate a physical, chemical or biological quantity into an electrical signal [28]. The transduction effect then allows electronics designers to access the information present in the real world parameters. By using a magnetic transducer, a system can measure the position of a fixed magnet (information) by producing an electrical signal analogue to the magnetic field magnitude at the location of the transducer.

The volume limitations in IMS means that there are also restrictions on the size of the transducers. This has been solved, however, thanks to developments in the field of Microelectromechanical Systems (MEMS). The term MEMS refers to devices that are composed of structures whose dimensions are in the micrometre range. MEMS are not limited only to silicon-based devices, and therefore nowadays, it is possible to find MEMS implemented in plastics, ceramics, and biological compounds [29], among other materials.

One of the first MEMS devices developed and commercialised are pressure sensors. These sensors are useful for numerous applications in the fields of industrial processes, automotive industry, consumer electronics, and biomedicine, to name a few. A pressure sensing MEMS element is usually based on a flexible membrane that can be deformed by force applied perpendicularly to its surface. The transducer then translates the strain on the material into an electrical parameter change, which then can be read by an electronic circuit. Depending on the application, a designer can choose among three types of sensors [30]:

- **Absolute pressure sensors:** the measurement is relative to vacuum. In this case, one side of the membrane is sealed closed to vacuum, while the other side is exposed to the medium. If the open end is vented to the atmosphere, then the reading is equal to the local atmospheric pressure (in average one bar or approximately 750 mmHg).

- **Gauge (Relative) pressure sensors:** the measurement is relative to the atmospheric pressure. On these sensors, one side of the sensing element is open to the local atmospheric pressure, while the other end is vented to the medium under measurement. If the measuring end is also vented to the atmosphere, then the reading is equal to 0 mmHg.

- **Differential pressure sensors:** these type of sensors are used to measure the pressure difference between two different pressure points. In these sensors, each side of the measuring membrane is attached to a port that connects it to a different pressure source. Anytime there is a difference between the pressure sources, then the reading deviates from 0 mmHg.

In pressure sensing, capacitive and piezoresistive MEMS transducers are the most common options on the market as well as in research. Each transduction method has advantages and disadvantages, which will be explored.

3.1.1 Piezoresistive pressure transducers

A large proportion of the MEMS pressure sensors available in the market are based on the piezoresistive effect. On these devices, a diaphragm is deformed due to the applied pressure. The deformation produces stress on piezoresistive elements placed on it. The applied strain is translated to a resistance change, which in turn can be then transformed into a variation of voltage or current.

The piezoresistive effect in silicon material was mentioned for the first time in a paper from Charles Smith from Bell Labs in 1954 [31]. Further developments lead to the invention of the first piezoresistive pressure sensors as in [32] and [33]. Nowadays, the piezoresistive effect, besides pressure sensing, is also used for accelerometers, cantilever force sensors, and inertial sensors [34].

The proportion of change $\Delta R_{\mathrm{pzr}}/R_{\mathrm{pzr}}$ in resistance for a given piezoresistive element is given by [35]:

$$\frac{\Delta R_{\mathrm{pzr}}}{R_{\mathrm{pzr}}} = (1+2\nu)\gamma_{\mathrm{s}} + \frac{\Delta\rho}{\rho}, \tag{3.1}$$

where ν is the material Poisson's ratio, γ_{s} is strain, and ρ is resistivity. From this equation, it is clear that the element resistance change is a result of the strain-induced change of the ratio between its cross-section and its longitudinal dimension (a geometric change of the element), as well as a fractional change on its resistivity $\Delta\rho/\rho$. When silicon is used as the material for the sensing element, the variation in resistivity is 50 to 100 times larger than the resistance variation induced by the geometric changes (i.e. elasticity) [35]. The direction of the stress or strain applied, as well as the direction of the current or electrical potential applied to the semiconductor element affect the observed piezoresistivity and elasticity [35].

Since its invention, the typical structure for a piezoresistive pressure sensor is based on placing four piezoresistors in a full Wheatstone bridge as in Fig.

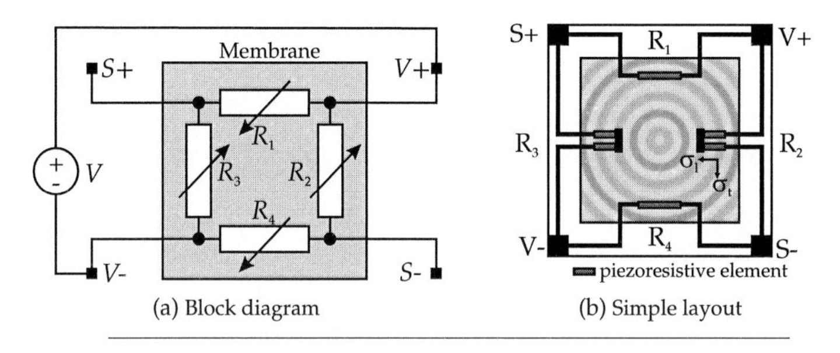

FIGURE 3.1: Piezoresistive pressure sensor: (a) diagram of the Wheatstone bridge resistor-array in a pressure sensor; (b) Simplified layout of a pressure sensor and the stress vectors (σ_l, σ_t) applied to R_2; on both figures V+ and V- are the supply voltage terminals, while S+ and S- are the bridge output terminals.

3.1.a. The elements are located as close as possible to the areas with maximum stress levels when pressure is applied to the membrane. An appropriate location and orientation of the elements increases the sensitivity and minimises the mismatch. In this way, two elements can be placed so that they are exposed to tensile stress, while the other pair is exposed to compressive forces. This arrangement results in the resistance increase of two sensing units while the other two units experience a reduction in resistance. The bridge voltage is proportional to the deformation of the measuring membrane when the units are in such a configuration [36].

In the case of the piezoresistive pressure sensor in Fig. 3.1.a and when applying a constant voltage V in the supply ports, the output voltage observed at its output is given by [34]:

$$V_{\text{bridge}} = S^+ - S^- = \frac{R_2 R_3 - R_1 R_4}{(R_1 + R_3)(R_2 + R_4)} V \tag{3.2}$$

Fig. 3.1.b shows the two stress components experienced by R_2 due to the pressure applied in the membrane. In this case, (σ_l) is the stress experienced on its longitudinal dimension, while (σ_t) is the stress on the transversal direction. Also, these two components are the same stress forces seen by R_3. In the case of R_1 and R_4, these components are rotated by 90 degrees, so for these resistors, the longitudinal stress is σ_t, and the transversal component is σ_l. Then, given these stress components, the resistance change ratio on each resistor is given by [34]:

$$\frac{\Delta R_2}{R_2} = -\frac{\Delta R_3}{R_3} = \alpha_1 = \pi_l \sigma_l + \pi_t \sigma_t \tag{3.3}$$

$$\frac{\Delta R_1}{R_1} = \frac{\Delta R_4}{R_4} = -\alpha_2 = \pi_l \sigma_t + \pi_t \sigma_l, \tag{3.4}$$

where π_t and π_l are the piezoresistive coefficients of silicon on the transversal and longitudinal directions, respectively. The values of α_1 and α_2 are positive. Then in the case of p-type piezoresistors (higher coefficients than n-type), the output voltage of the transducer can be approximated to [34, 37]:

$$V_{\text{bridge}} = \frac{V}{2} \pi_{44} \left| \sigma_y - \sigma_x \right|, \tag{3.5}$$

which shows that the output voltage depends on the stress resulting from the membrane deformation (and the piezoresistive coefficient of silicon π_{44}). Thus a linear relationship with the applied pressure is obtained.

3.1.2 Capacitive pressure transducers

Capacitive transducers operation principle is the change in their electrical capacitance. Fig. 3.2 shows a representation of the different mechanisms that lead to a change in capacitance in a capacitive transducer [38]. In the case of sensing of mechanical parameters, such as pressure, using the change in the distance between plates as a transduction method (Fig. 3.2.a) provides the best sensitivity. However, due to non-linearity, it is limited to small ranges. In the case of needing a broader dynamic range, as in displacement measurements, using the capacitor area change as in Fig. 3.2.b (caused by the movement of one of the plates while the distance between plates is constant), provides good linearity with the penalty of decreasing the sensitivity.

Another sensing method is the variation of the relative permittivity ϵ of the dielectric as in Figure 3.2.c. The permittivity change is the result of applying force to the dielectric, or absorption of chemicals or moisture from the medium. This sensing method is used in chemical sensors [38]. A fourth sensing method consists of detecting changes in the properties of one of the electrodes, as in Figure 3.2.d. A typical example of this kind of sensors are capacitive touch screens, where the finger touching the glass screen acts as one of the plates of a capacitor (the other electrode resides below the glass screen).

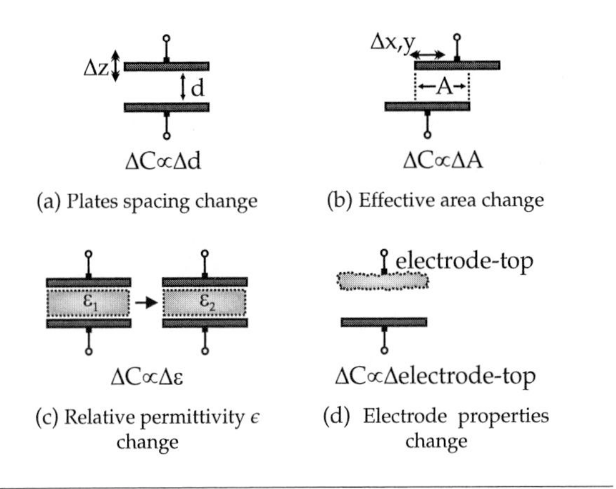

FIGURE 3.2: Transduction mechanisms in a capacitive sensor: The capacitance value can vary due to changes in (a) spacing between plates, (b) effective area, (c) dielectric relative permittivity, (d) geometry and electrical properties of an electrode.

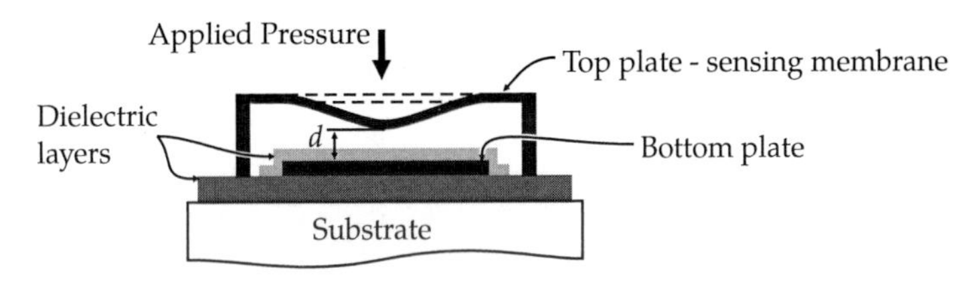

FIGURE 3.3: Simplified cross-section of a capacitive pressure sensing element.

In the particular case of miniature capacitive pressure sensors, the sensing is based on the deformation of a membrane as in [39, 40, 41, 42], which is similar to piezoresistive pressure sensors. However, the electrical parameter change (i.e. capacitance) seen by the readout hardware is not caused by the deformation of the membrane element (as in the case of the piezoresistive transducer) but by its displacement when pressure is applied. Figure 3.3 shows a simplified cross-section view of a thin-film capacitive pressure element; it is possible to note the effect of pressure on the sensing membrane and how it produces a change in the distance d between the plates.

As can be observed in Figure 3.3, when applying pressure, the top plate is not displaced, but it experiences a deflection. The ratio of capacitance change is therefore dependent on the geometry (shape, dimensions and thickness) of the membrane, as well as on its material properties, such as its Poisson's ratio ν (how much it compresses or expands due to a load) and Young's modulus E (the relationship between strain and stress for the material). As a result, the change in capacitance for a generic membrane geometry can be calculated as [43]:

$$v = \frac{1}{A} \int_{y_{\min}}^{y_{\max}} \int_{x_{\min}}^{x_{\max}} \omega(x, y, P) \, \mathrm{d}x \, \mathrm{d}y \tag{3.6}$$

$$\Delta C = C_0 \left(\frac{v}{d_0 - v} \right), \tag{3.7}$$

where v is is the mean displacement of the top membrane electrode, A is the electrode area, d_0 is the resting position distance between electrodes, and ω is the deflection experienced as a function of the applied pressure (the membrane geometry and material properties define this function) at coordinates (x, y). For instance, the capacitance change ΔC produced by the pressure P applied to the sensor in [44], which is designed using a round (with a radius a) miniature thin-film membrane as sensing element, is given by:

$$\omega(r, P) = \frac{3Pa(1 - \nu^2)}{8Eh^3} \left(r^2 - a^2 \right)^2 \tag{3.8}$$

$$\Delta C(P) = \int_0^a \epsilon \frac{2r}{z - \omega(r, P)} \, \mathrm{d}r - C_0, \tag{3.9}$$

As presented, the change in capacitance has a non-linear relationship with the pressure; however, a linear approximation can be obtained for displacements that are small compared with the thickness of the membrane [43]. Maintaining a minimized displacement means that the dynamic pressure range on these transducers is limited, but their sensitivity can be higher than that achieved with piezoresistive sensors. Also, the temperature dependency and long-term stability of these sensors present better results when compared to their piezoresistive counterparts [43, 45]. Furthermore, capacitive transducers are suitable for high-pressure applications since the substrate acts as an over-pressure protection [39].

3.2 Data acquisition

The main task for an implantable monitoring system is to process a physical parameter (such as pressure) and transform it into an electrical signal (or other variable) that can be measured and converted to a digital value that can be stored and transmitted electrically [46]. Figure 3.4 presents a conceptual diagram of the data acquisition process. This diagram depicts a generic flow which covers three domains: physical, electrical and digital. On each level, different error sources are present. These error sources have to be accounted for by the designer so that the information presented to the application layer (e.g. the user: a physician) represents the reality with a sufficient level of accuracy (dictated by the application) that the physical phenomena under observation can be properly interpreted.

The complexity of the hardware used to acquire the data is then dependent on the level of precision and accuracy required by the application. The typical methodology used is to define a noise budget along the information conversion path. For this, every source of noise has to be identified. Then, based on the requirements for resolution for the whole system, it is possible to determine the acceptable error contribution on each stage. With this information, the designer can then decide the design specifications and parameters for each functional block in the acquisition system.

Some of the error sources in Figure 3.4 can be reduced at the circuit level as the electrical noise in the front-end amplifiers. Some errors as thermal drift in the transducer require an architectural solution (the system would need to measure also the temperature to apply a compensation algorithm). Any error introduced after the data conversion stage is not discussed in this work.

3.2.1 Piezoresistive pressure sensor signal path

In Section 3.1.1 piezoresistive pressure sensors were introduced and described. Equation 3.2 showed that when placing four piezoresistive elements in a Wheatstone bridge configuration, the changes in resistance are translated to a variation in the voltage value V_{bridge} between the output nodes of the transducer array. In this way, the piezoresistive transducer unit works as a pressure-to-resistance-to-voltage converter (the first stage of the signal path presented in Figure 3.5). In the same data path and the downstream direction, a conditioning stage is required to take the output of the transducer and convert it to a more suitable signal for digitising, this is a voltage-to-voltage

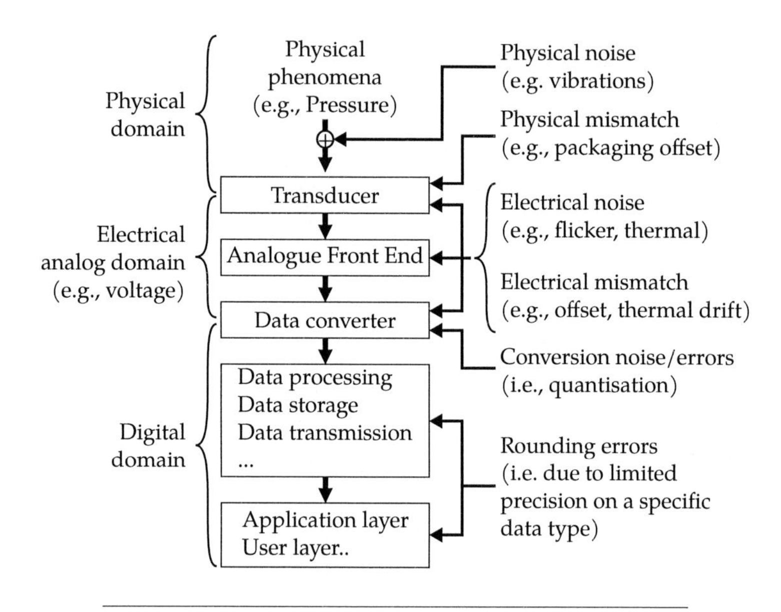

FIGURE 3.4: Conceptual diagram of the data acquisition process (including some error sources).

conversion ($V_{sAFE}(V_{bridge})$). Therefore, the task of this analogue front-end is to amplify and filter the signal. An N-bit ADC then digitises the output of this conditioning stage.

Each of the blocks shown in Figure 3.5also represents a noise source that has to be accounted to determine whether the data-path output provides useful information to detect the variations of pressure at its input. Therefore, a noise budget analysis can be used to determine the design parameters for each of the blocks involved in the data path.

3.2.1.1 Noise analysis

Figure 3.6 shows the noise sources affecting the signal path when using the piezoresistive transducer. As mentioned earlier, the noise budget on the system can be used to define the requirements of each stage. In this section, such analysis is done for a generic interface.

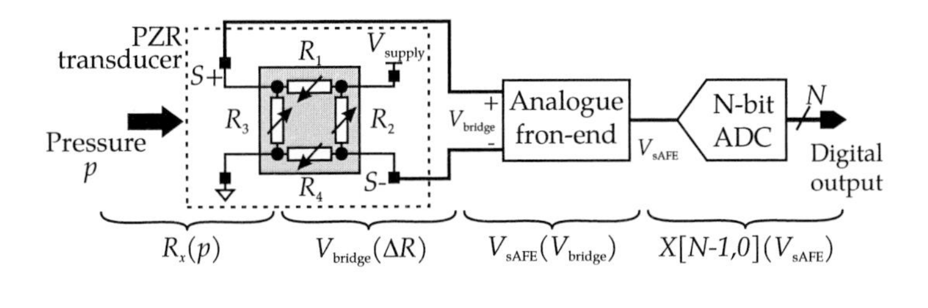

FIGURE 3.5: Simplified block diagram of a piezoresistive readout interface.

Noise contribution from the piezoresistive element

As shown in Figure 3.6, several sources of noise are related to the sensing element. A list of these sources and the mechanisms that generate such noise is presented:

- **1/f (Hooge) noise:** Also known as pink or flicker noise, this is a noise whose magnitude is inversely proportional to the frequency. Some models attribute this noise to bulk defects that cause fluctuations in the number of carriers or their mobility. In a piezoresistive element, the pink noise is due to conductivity fluctuations in the resistors, and no current is required to generate it, however since it is a variation in the conductance, current is required to observe its effect [47]. Given the behaviour of this noise source, the uncertainty contribution added to a sampled acquired depends on the measurement bandwidth. The $1/f$ noise for a single sensing element (resistor) is given by [47]:

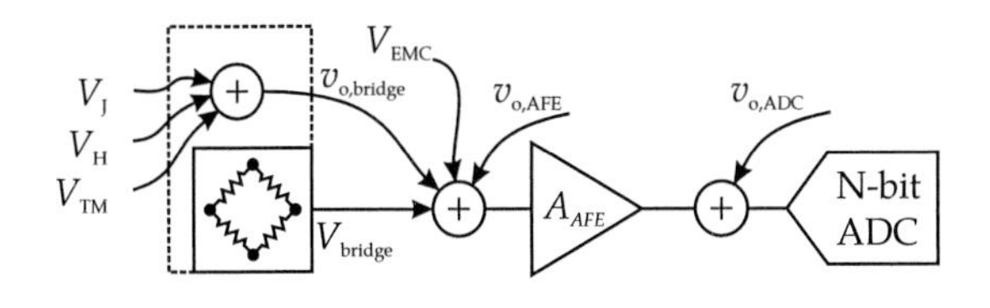

FIGURE 3.6: Noise sources in the piezoresistive pressure sensor data-path: Johnson Noise V_J, $1/f$ noise (Hooge) V_H, thermo-mechanical noise V_{TM}, electromagnetic coupling noise V_{EMC}, analogue front-end $v_{o,AFE}$ and ADC $v_{o,ADC}$ noise (quantisation).

$$V_{\mathrm{H}} = \frac{V_{\mathrm{bridge}}}{2} \sqrt{\frac{\alpha}{N_{\mathrm{eff}}} \ln \frac{f_{\max}}{f_{\min}}}, \tag{3.10}$$

where α is a non-dimensional fitting parameter that depends on the fabrication process; $f_{\max}$ and $f_{\min}$ define the measuring frequency band, and N_{eff} is the effective number of carriers of the piezoresistive element. As per this relationship, the $1/f$ noise can only be improved by selecting the appropriate measurement bandwidth or by optimisations in the fabrication of the sensing element (this work was limited to a commercially available device, so this level of design was not explored). For low-frequency applications, this noise source can tend to dominate or become significant [48].

- **Johnson (thermal) noise:** The thermal agitation of atoms causes the thermal noise or Johnson noise (in honour of its first observation by J.B. Johnson in 1928 [46]). This electrical noise has its source on the random movement of mobile carriers in electrically resistive materials [47, 48]. The noise power spectral density is independent of the frequency and exists on any device or element that posses electrical resistivity. By integrating the power spectral density of the thermal noise over the measurement bandwidth ($f_{\max} - f_{\min}$), the RMS Johnson voltage noise can be calculated as [47]:

$$V_{\mathrm{J}} = \sqrt{4k_{\mathrm{B}}TR_{\mathrm{pzr}}(f_{\max} - f_{\min})}, \tag{3.11}$$

where T is the temperature of the resistor with resistance R_{pzr}. Since the resistance of the commercially available sensor cannot be changed, and T is the internal body temperature (for the IMS application), the only optimisation can be done in the measurement bandwidth. This noise becomes important when the voltage resolution in the sensor is close to the thermal voltage [48].

- **Thermomechanical noise:** This noise becomes important for systems where the technology is used on its limits [49]. Also known as Brownian noise, its source is common to Johnson noise since it is based on the relationship between temperature and the vibration of atoms, yet, in this case, the nature of the noise is mechanical. This noise is important for miniaturised very thin membranes [48]. Small parts in modern sensors are highly susceptible to mechanical noise due to molecular agitation; hence its amplitude depends on the force sensitivity of the transducer (S_{FV}, in V N^{-1} units) [47]. In the case of pressure sensing, the equivalent mechanical noise is in the range of 10^{-9} mmHg [50]. As with the Johnson noise, the power spectral density of the thermomechanical noise is independent on the frequency. From this, the RMS noise voltage in a measurement bandwidth given by $f_{\max} - f_{\min}$, is computed as [47]:

$$V_{TM} = S_{FV}\sqrt{\frac{4k_B T}{\omega_0 Q}(f_{\max} - f_{\min})}. \tag{3.12}$$

Given these noise sources, the total RMS noise contribution from the pressure transducer seen at the input of the analogue front end can be calculated as the superposition of each noise source [48]:

$$v_{o,\mathrm{bridge}} = \sqrt{V_H^2 + V_J^2 + V_{TM}^2}\,, \tag{3.13}$$

the weight of each one of these components depends on the application and the characteristics of the specific transducer. In the case of the present work, the thermomechanical component can be assumed negligible since the target resolution is in the range of 10^{-1} mmHg. Also, the jitter noise ($1/f$) can be reduced by averaging the output over the sampling interval [50]. Then the noise from the transceiver can be approximated to only the thermal (Johnson) noise.

Aside from these noise sources that act directly on the transducer unit, the electromagnetic coupling noise can be present when there is improper shielding or when the system is surrounded by strong fields. This interference has to be accounted for during design in order to reduce its impact. Good practices on PCB and routing design, as well as keeping the transducer as close as possible to the electronics helps to reduce the coupling of undesired electromagnetic signals.

Noise contribution from the analogue front-end

The Analogue front-end (AFE) used to condition the small-signal received from the transducer can be as simple as a single operational amplifier, or as complex as a multistage system with several amplifiers, active filters and switched networks as a chopper stage. Independently of the design of the AFE, the typical methodology is that the first amplification stage noise represents the dominant noise contribution in the data path [47]. A typical case for piezoresistive sensors in a Wheatstone bridge configuration is to use an instrumentation amplifier as the first stage.

In a CMOS front-end system the typical error sources are offset, drift, $1/f$ noise and thermal noise. Figure 3.7 shows these error sources on a typical AFE noise PSD. As shown, the dominant errors depend on the bandwidth and centre frequency required by the application. The sensing operation in the present work has a low bandwidth, and therefore the $1/f$ noise is dominant together with the offset and drift errors.

Low-frequency errors such as offset, drift, and $1/f$ noise can be reduced by using dynamic circuit techniques as auto-zeroing, chopping or fixed solutions as trimming. A typical selection for the stage for an AFE is an instrumentation amplifier. In this construction block, both, $1/f$ and thermal noise contribution from the amplifier are in both current and voltage. By calculating the voltage and current coefficients of the $1/f$ (A_{VF} and A_{IF}, respectively) and thermal (A_{VJ} and A_{IJ}, respectively) noise, it is possible to determine the integrated RMS voltage noise from the front-end [47]:

$$v_{\mathrm{o,AFE}} = \left[\left[A_{\mathrm{VJ}}^2 + 2A_{\mathrm{IJ}}^2\left(\frac{R_{\mathrm{pzr}}}{2}\right)^2\right](f_{\mathrm{max}} - f_{\mathrm{min}}) + \left[A_{\mathrm{VF}}^2 + 2A_{\mathrm{IF}}^2\left(\frac{R_{\mathrm{pzr}}}{2}\right)^2\right]\ln\left(\frac{f_{\mathrm{max}}}{f_{\mathrm{min}}}\right)\right]^{\frac{1}{2}} \tag{3.14}$$

This relationship shows that the design of the first amplification stage in the AFE has to take into account the characteristics of the transceiver in the system in order to get the best solution for reaching the target system signal-to-noise ratio and resolution.

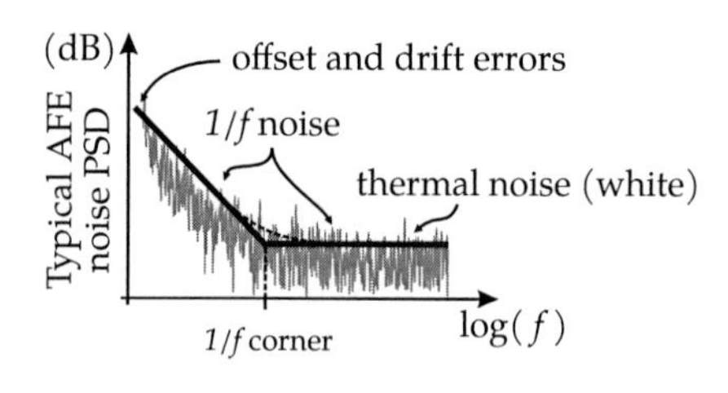

FIGURE 3.7: Noise profile on an analogue front-end

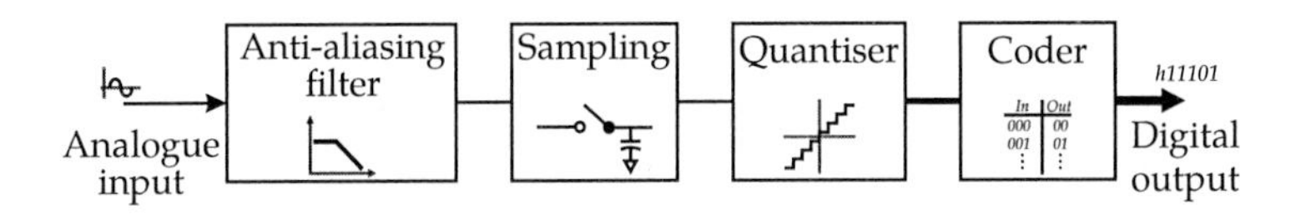

FIGURE 3.8: Basic block diagram with the basic elements in an ADC

Noise contribution from the analogue-to-digital converter

The final stage on the piezoresistive sensor data-path is the analogue to digital conversion. Figure 3.8 shows the essential elements that interact in a typical ADC. As in the case of the upper-level system view of the data-path (Figure 3.6), each element adds noise and errors to the output. As in the previous two blocks, the most critical error sources are described for a generic implementation in order to understand the role they play regarding the final system resolution.

- **Jitter noise:** In the sampling phase, the system is prone to add errors due to jitter. The added noise has as main source the any period variation in the system clock (jitter) and uncertainties in the delays through the logic used to control the different switches that conform the sampling block [51]. This source of error is widely known as phase noise. Figure 3.9 shows a depiction of the mechanism that leads to error. The timing jitter is normally assumed as a white noise. The uncertainty of the sampling time due to the jitter causes a variation on the sampled voltage that has a high dependency on the first derivative of the input signal ($f(t)$ in Figure 3.9). The error probability errors are then linearly scaled by the slope of the signal around the ideal sampling time. For a given clock jitter, the effect of this phenomena is larger in faster input signals

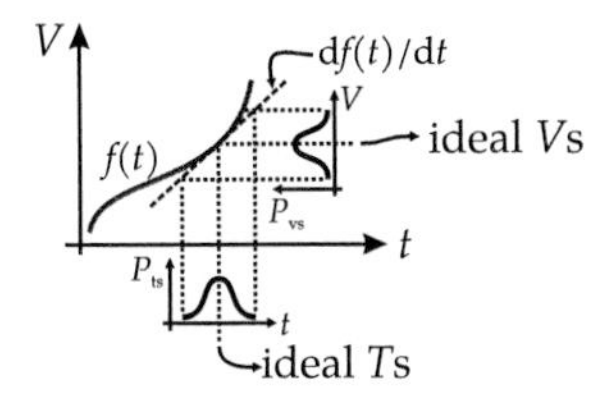

FIGURE 3.9: Phase noise action mechanism.

(higher slope) than for low-frequency inputs. In this way, for a sinusoidal signal input with amplitude V_0 and frequency f_0, the RMS voltage error introduced by a total jitter t_j is given by [52]:

$$V_{\text{jitter}} = \frac{2\pi f_0 V_0 t_j}{\sqrt{2}} \quad (3.15)$$

- **Quantisation noise:** Another ADC intrinsic error source is the quantisation noise. After successfully sampling the signal, the quantiser maps the continuous range of amplitudes of the samples into a set of finite output codes. For this task the full range of possible input values V_{FR} is divided into the number of discrete values in the output set M:

$$V_{\text{LSB}} = \frac{V_{\text{FR}}}{M}, \quad (3.16)$$

this value is the step size and ideally is constant for all the valid input range. Figure 3.10 shows a simplified view of the quantisation error. As can be seen, the maximum magnitude for the error is $V_{\text{LSB}}/2$, which occurs on the transitions between steps.

A detailed analysis of this noise source shows that there is some correlation between the input signal properties and the quantisation noise. However, a good approximation for the RMS quantisation noise component can be calculated by integrating the error signal (shown in the figure) as [52]:

$$V_{\text{quantisation}} = \frac{V_{\text{LSB}}}{\sqrt{12}}. \quad (3.17)$$

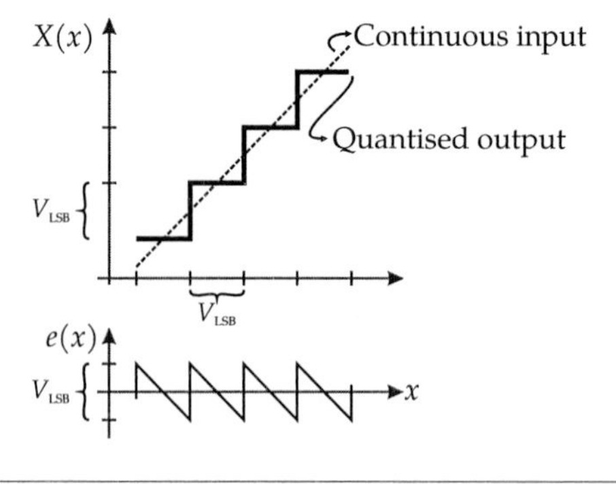

FIGURE 3.10: Quantisation noise concept.

- **Thermal noise:** The quantisation noise described previously is always present in data converters and represents a limit to the performance of the device. The quantisation noise is inherent to the functionality of data converters, yet another source related to the physical nature of the circuits used for ADCs leads to further limitations of the system: thermal noise. As described for the transceiver and the AFE, thermal or kT/C noise is always present in any electronic component due to the random vibrations of atoms. For an ADC, this source of noise is independent of the characteristics of the input signal (e.g. shape, amplitude or frequency) [52]. As described in [51], this error source results from noise integrated in the sampling capacitance in the system and its RMS value is calculated as:

$$V_{\mathrm{thermal}} = \sqrt{\frac{k_{\mathrm{B}}T}{C_{\mathrm{s}}}} \,. \tag{3.18}$$

The description of these three noise sources added in the ADC stage, together with the system level resolution and noise budget requirements, can be used to define the design parameters for its different components. Furthermore, the mentioned definitions are used as criteria to select the appropriate architecture for the ADC.

3.2.1.2 Piezoresistive sensor interface implementation

Figure 3.5 shows the minimum system required to digitise the output of a piezoresistive transducer. As described in the previous section, the specifications from each block depends on the noise budget set to achieve the target resolution. Therefore each block can be defined from the total noise goals. The total noise expected, for the minimum piezoresistive interface (Figure 3.5), can be calculated at the ADC input as:

$$N_{\mathrm{o,sys}} = N_{\mathrm{o,bridge}} * A_{\mathrm{AFE}}^2 + N_{\mathrm{o,AFE}} + N_{\mathrm{o,ADC}} \,, \tag{3.19}$$

The maximum uncertainty allowed in the output (noise budget) can be expressed as the relationship between the transducer sensitivity S_{pzr}, the bridge supply voltage $V_{\mathrm{dd,bridge}}$ and the expected resolution (p_{r}):

$$N_{\mathrm{o,sys,max}} = \left(\frac{S_{\mathrm{pzr}} V_{\mathrm{dd,bridge}} p_{\mathrm{r}}}{\alpha} \right)^2 , \tag{3.20}$$

where α is the deviation factor (α equal to six accounts for 99.7% of errors). By defining the noise budget and assigning weights (W_x) to the noise contribution from each element in the signal path, it is possible to define the maximum noise that is allowed to be introduced on each stage. In this way, by using Equation 3.19:

$$W_{\text{bridge}} + W_{\text{AFE}} + W_{\text{ADC}} = 1 \,, \tag{3.21}$$

$$N_{\text{o,sys,max}} W_{\text{bridge}} = N_{\text{o,bridge}} * A^2_{\text{AFE}} \,, \tag{3.22}$$

$$N_{\text{o,sys,max}} W_{\text{AFE}} = N_{\text{o,AFE}} \,, \tag{3.23}$$

$$N_{\text{o,sys,max}} W_{\text{ADC}} = N_{\text{o,ADC}} \,. \tag{3.24}$$

With these equations, a noise budget value, and the relationships that define the sources on each stage (Section 3.2.1.1) it is possible to determine the design parameters for the entire signal path. In a simplified interface model that only considers the thermal noise and the quantisation noise, the uncertainty added by each stage is given by:

$$N_{\text{o,bridge}} = 4k_{\text{B}} T R_{\text{bridge}} B_{\text{bridge}} A_{\text{AFE}} \,, \tag{3.25}$$

$$N_{\text{o,AFE}} = S_{\text{n,in,v,AFE}} B_{\text{AFE}} A_{\text{AFE}} = V^2_{\text{n,in,AFE}} A_{\text{AFE}} \,, \tag{3.26}$$

$$N_{\text{o,ADC}} = \frac{1}{12} V^2_{\text{REF}} 2^{-2b} \,, \tag{3.27}$$

where $S_{\text{n,in,v,AFE}}$ and $V_{\text{n,in,AFE}}$ are the AFE input-referred noise spectrum density and noise voltage, respectively. Furthermore, B_{bridge} is the piezoresistor bandwidth calculated as $B_{\text{bridge}} = (2\pi R_{\text{bridge}} C_{\text{in,AFE}})^{-1}$ ($C_{\text{in,AFE}}$ is the AFE input capacitance seen by the bridge). Moreover, the effective piezoresistor bandwidth is approximated to the AFE bandwidth by meeting the condition $B_{\text{bridge}} > B_{\text{AFE}}$.

The relations from Equation 3.20 to Equation 3.27 define the trade-off between the different specifications for the AFE and ADC. As seen on these relationships, the selection of a specific piezoresistive transducer affects the overall system. With the target system requirements and the characteristics of the sensing element, it is possible to define its interface.

During the evaluation of piezoresistive transducers for this project, two interfaces were developed. The first interface was based on elements from the analogue library from AMS-AG (Austria Mikro Systeme). This first implementation was realised to provide an on-chip interface for the initial test of piezoresistive elements. The second implementation is still a work on progress and aims to achieve resolution as high as 0.1 mmHg of pressure.

SAR-based test interface in 350 nm CMOS technology

The test ASIC in Appendix B.1 included an interface to evaluate the use of piezoresistive pressure sensors. Figure 3.11.a shows the block diagram of the implemented interface. For the development of this interface, elements from the AMS analogue library were used. These devices are of general purpose and are not optimised for our area or ultra-low-power operation requirements; however, this interface provided a vehicle for initial tests and prototyping. As displayed, the AFE is implemented by an instrumentation amplifier. For this implementation, low noise amplifiers were used. As shown, the amplifier gain is controlled by an external resistor R_G which provides flexibility to adjust it at a system level.

The design makes use of a 10-bit SAR-ADC for the digitisation of the conditioned transducer output value. A 1MHz clock for this unit is provided

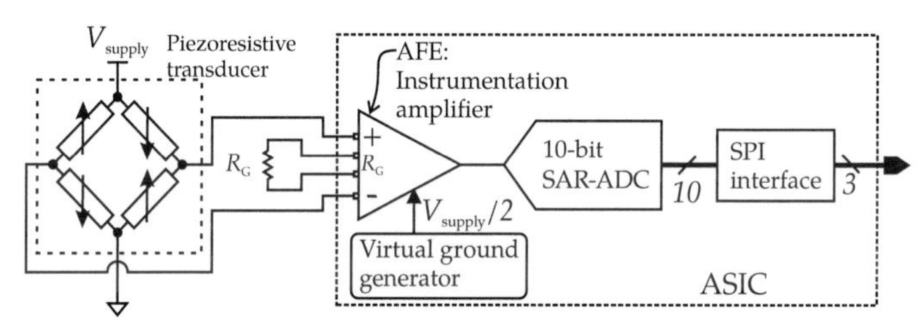

(a) Block diagram of the implemented piezoresistive pressure sensor interface.

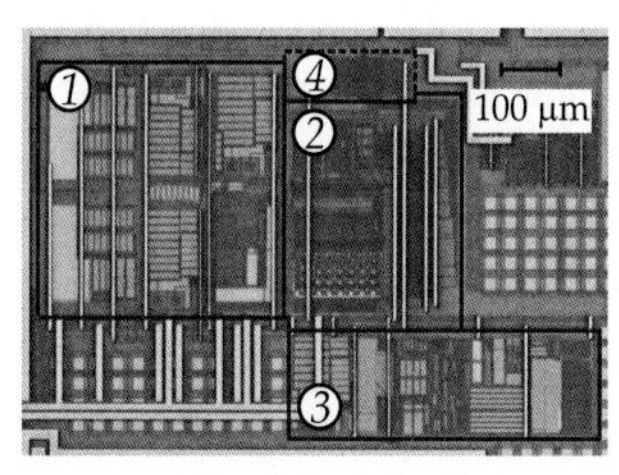

(b) Annotated micrograph of the piezoresistive interface implemented in 350 nm CMOS technology. 1. Analogue front-end, 2. 10-bits SAR-ADC, 3. Virtual ground circuit, 4. SPI interface (test only).

FIGURE 3.11: Piezoresistive pressure sensor interface implemented in AMS 350 nm CMOS technology.

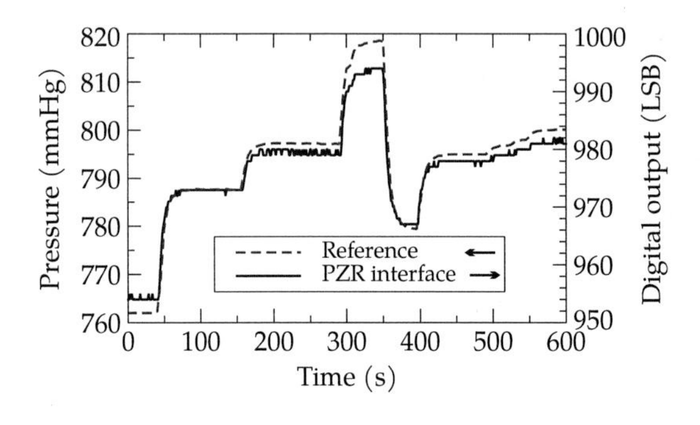

FIGURE 3.12: Digital output value for the first piezoresistive interface.

externally. The output from this unit consists of the 10 bits of data and an End-Of-Conversion (EOC) signal. As shown in Figure 3.11.a, the data output lines from the ADC are connected to an SPI interface. This SPI unit is not an integral part of the described piezoresistive sensor interface and is only used for test purposes. The SPI block serialises the ADC output to use only three pads from the test ASIC (instead of the ten pads required if using the ADC directly).

An annotated micrograph of the implemented interface is shown in Figure 3.11.b. The total area used by this unit was $0.35\,\mathrm{mm}^2$. The power consumption of the system during operation (the device is disconnected from the supply when not used) was in average 4.95 mW.

This interface was tested by using a commercially available piezoresistive pressure transducer [53]. By using the test chamber in Appendix C, several steps of pressure were applied to the sensing device to verify the functionality. Figure 3.12 presents a test run on this piezoresistive interface. The graph shows the applied pressure measured by the reference system (dotted line), and the uncompensated digital output from the ADC.

Definition of a fully custom interface in 180 nm CMOS technology

The power and area consumption from the previously presented interface requires optimisation to be a candidate component for miniaturised semi-autonomous IMS. Therefore, the development of a fully custom interface concept was started during this work. The piezoresistive sensor selected for the future implantable system has a bridge resistance of 5.81 kΩ and has a sensitivity of $36.0 \pm 7.2\,\mu V\,mmHg^{-1}$ at 1.8 V supply voltage. Also, as a system specification, the maximum pressure variation expected is 350 mmHg with a resolution of 0.1 mmHg.

By calculating Equation 3.20 using the system-level specifications, and assuming a reference voltage of 1.6V at the amplifier, the noise budget for the system becomes $N_{o,sys,max} = 5.805 \times 10^{-9} V^2$. From this value, the design equations presented in this section, and using numeric methods, it was possible to define the front-end and ADC requirements to achieve the expected pressure resolution (0.1 mmHg). The AFE design requires a gain of 35 and a maximum integrated noise of 2.134 µV (with a bandwidth of 1.43 kHz). Finally, it was defined that a 16 bits ADC is required for this system.

Given these specifications, this work focused on preparing an initial design for the ADC. The ADC selection was based on the required bit-resolution (16 bits), the need for noise reduction and that speed is not an obstacle since the application sampling rate is in the milli-hertz range. Due to these criteria, an Incremental Sigma-Delta ADC (IΣΔADC) is proposed [54].

Sigma-delta ADC are widely used in applications that require high-resolution analogue to digital conversions. In particular, the use of IΣΔADC is a good option for low-frequency applications where high-resolution is essential. Furthermore, this type of converter can be easily multiplexed and offers more straightforward decimation filtering [55].

As with any sigma-delta ADC, IΣΔADC consists of two main blocks: a sigma-delta modulator and a digital filter. However, the IΣΔADC differs from other sigma-delta ADC on the way it digitises its analogue input. The conversion process on an IΣΔADC is started after a reset that clears the digital and analogue memory elements. After the reset, the system performs the conversion taking N clock cycles (at which the modulator generates a bitstream that is processed by the digital filters to produce the digital output). The conversion ends with saving the module output value and a new reset. In this way, the IΣΔADC performs the conversion in a sample by sample fashion, therefore working as a Nyquist-rate analogue-to-digital converter [55].

As part of this initial step to provide a custom interface for piezoresistive sensors, it was decided to implement the modulator for the IΣΔADC on a test ASIC, while leaving the design of the digital filter for a second design stage once the modulator has been optimised. In this way, the design efforts are firstly focused on optimising the analogue blocks related to the modulator. Additionally, having a Sigma-Delta Modulator (ΣΔM) in hardware brings flexibility to the design and debug tasks for the digital filters, since an FPGA can be used together with the ASIC.

Since ΣΔM are widely used, the literature presents a large variety of implementations. However, the primary variations on the architectures are [56]:

- Number of quantisers: Those devices using only one quantiser are known as single-loop topologies. ΣΔM with more than one quantiser are denominated cascade or multiloop sigma-delta modulators. Cascade ΣΔM solve the stability problems present in high-order single-loop ΣΔM; however, their area and power consumption are higher.
- Number of bits in the quantiser: Most ΣΔM use a one-bit quantiser. However, some architectures make use of multi-bit quantisers, which can provide some advantages. Each additional bit on the quantiser gets a reduction close to 6dB on the quantisation noise. Furthermore, the stability of multi-bit ΣΔM is better than its single-bit counterparts. However, the use of quantisers with multiple bits requires more circuitry and adds more dependency to process mismatch.
- Circuit techniques used: The implementation of the ΣΔM can be done using continuous-time or discrete-time circuit techniques. Until recently, most implementations were based on discrete-time ΣΔM; however, the need for higher sampling rates has attracted the attention to continuous-time SDM. The main difference between these two categories is the location of the sampling in the ΣΔM loop. For a discrete-time ΣΔM, the sampling circuitry is located at its input, allowing to use discrete circuits for the complete module. Differently, continuous-time ΣΔM places the sampling unit before the quantiser, meaning that most of the blocks in the loop are design following continuous-time techniques.
- Loop order: The accuracy of a ΣΔ-ADC is improved by increasing the noise shaping order since it shifts more quantisation noise out of the band of interest. However, orders larger than two could lead to stability issues.
- Oversampling ratio: As higher the Oversampling Ratio (OSR), the better the ideal dynamic range of a ΣΔ-ADC; However, increasing the OSR results in higher sampling frequencies and therefore, higher dynamic

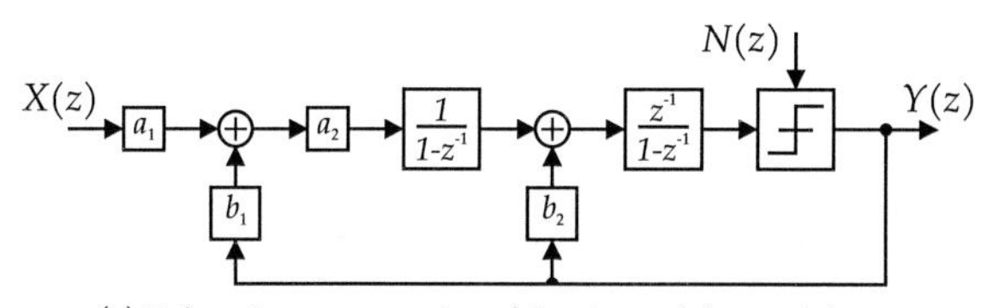

(a) Z domain representation of the sigma-delta modulator.

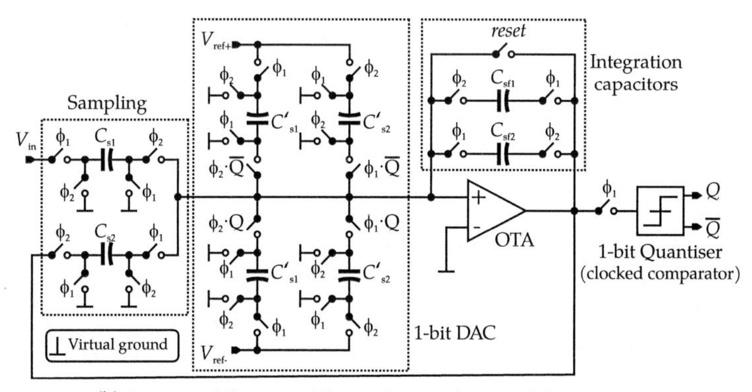

(b) Conceptual diagram of the implemented sigma-delta modulator.

FIGURE 3.13: Sigma-delta modulator implemented concept [57].

power consumption (when compared to a similar design with reduced OSR).

Based on the above theory and the target application, it was decided to design a single-loop second-order discrete-time ΣΔM for this work. By employing a second-order modulator, the number of cycles for a 16-bit conversion is reduced from 65536 to 512. A 2 MHz sampling frequency and oversampling ratio of 512 ensures that the ADC can process the already established bandwidth of 1.43 kHz (from AFE).

Figure 3.13.a shows the z-domain diagram for the proposed modulator. For this system, the signal and noise transfer functions are [57]:

$$STF(z) = \frac{a_1 a_2 z^{-1}}{1 + (a_2 b_1 + b_2 - 2)z^{-1} + (1 - b_2)z^{-2}}, \tag{3.28}$$

$$NTF(z) = \frac{(1 - z^{-1})^2}{1 + (a_2 b_1 + b_2 - 2)z^{-1} + (1 - b_2)z^{-2}} \tag{3.29}$$

respectively. The signal transfer function (STF) reveals the low-pass filtering nature of the modulator, while the noise transfer function (NTF) presents the high-pass effect, effectively shaping the noise out from the signal band. A direct implementation of the presented diagram (Figure 3.13.a) would require the use of two amplification stages. However, area savings are possible by multiplexing a single amplifier. Figure 3.13.b displays a schematic of the ΣΔM implemented using a single Operational Transconductance Amplifier [54, 57]. The capacitance values in the schematic are related to the transfer function coefficients by:

$$a_1 = \frac{C_{s1}}{C_{f1}}, \quad b_1 = \frac{C'_{s1}}{C_{f1}}, \quad a_2 = \frac{C_{s2}}{C_{f2}}, \quad b_2 = \frac{C'_{s2}}{C_{f2}}. \tag{3.30}$$

The coefficients (and the capacitance values) are calculated by maximising the modulator SNR. Furthermore, since the capacitance values directly affect the system area, a second criteria to define these values is on minimising the total capacitance (hence the area). The previous requires to explore the effective capacitance seen by the OTA during sampling and integration steps, which are given by:

$$C_{eff1} = (a_1 + b_1)C_{f1} + a_2(a_1 + b_1 + 1)C_{f2}, \tag{3.31}$$

$$C_{eff2} = (a_2 + b_2 + 1)C_{f2}. \tag{3.32}$$

The previous optimisation criteria assumes an ideal OTA. However, OTA non-idealities such as finite DC-gain, slew rate, saturation voltage, and gain bandwidth results in incomplete transfer of charge in the switched capacitor network, degrading the SNR of the ΣΔM. Also, the CMOS switches finite resistance, parasitic capacitors and mismatch contribute to the design degradation. Due to the mentioned performance loss, it is critical to determine the source of these non-idealities so that constraints for the OTA can be defined [58].

Based on the analysis presented and the system specifications, a prototype modulator was implemented in 180 nm CMOS technology [54]. The developed system integrated on-chip the switched capacitor network (sampling, 1-bit DAC and integration), the OTA, and the clocked comparator are shown in Figure 3.13.b. Moreover, the design also included the control circuitry for the switches and a non-overlapping clock generator. The switches were implemented as CMOS transmission gates that included dummy transistors to mitigate the charge injection effects [54, 59].

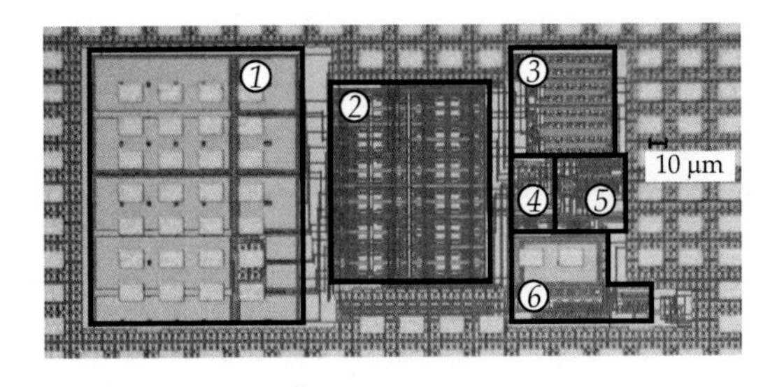

FIGURE 3.14: Annotated micrograph of the implemented ΣΔM in 180 nm CMOS technology. 1. Capacitor bank, 2. Switch array, 3. Non-overlapping clock generation, 4. Clock control, 5. Comparator, 6. OTA.

A functional prototype of this modulator was fabricated as part of the test ASIC shown in Appendix B.3 (The chip in Appendix B.2 also included the modulator; however a layout error lead to a deficient clock distribution), an annotated micrograph is displayed in Figure 3.14. The total area occupied by the modulator prototype is 0.058 mm^2.

The modulator was tested using an external 4 MHz clock (that sets a sampling time of 2 MHz). Figure 3.15 shows the resulting output spectral

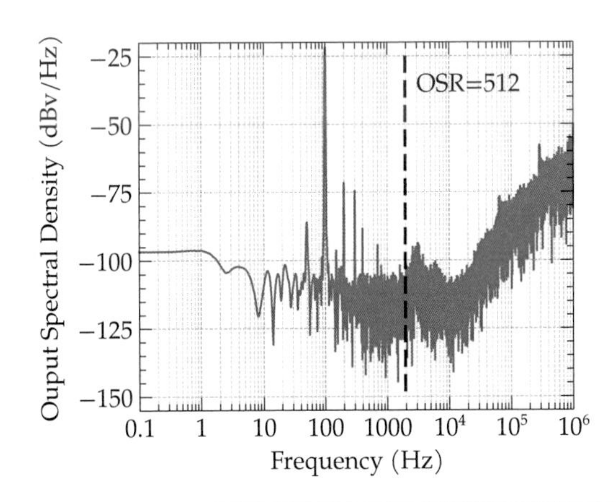

FIGURE 3.15: Power spectral density of the implemented sigma-delta modulator (input: 500 mVpp at 100 Hz, Virtual ground: 900 mV DC)

density for the modulator with a sinusoidal signal at the input. The resulting curve shows the expected noise shaping towards high frequencies. For this test, a sinusoidal signal with an amplitude of 250 mV and a frequency of 100 Hz was applied. In this case, and for an oversampling ratio of 512 (1.953 kHz bandwidth), the measured SNR is 58.39 dB, resulting in an ENOB of 9.4070 bits. The modulator uses on average 167.32 µW during operation.

The results obtained from this first version of sigma-delta modulator represent the first step towards a fully integrated interface for piezoresistive pressure sensors in our system. The results provide information for further improvements: the large harmonic spikes could have their root cause on the parasitic elements in the system. In this case, rerouting the system taking better care of parasitic elements can provide significant improvements [57].

3.2.2 Capacitive pressure sensor interface

As described in Section 3.1.2, capacitive pressure transducers are based on the deflection of a semi-flexible electrode when pressure is applied. The deflection causes variation on the distance between the flexible electrode and a fixed one, which in turn is reflected as a capacitance change. The readout circuitry used for capacitive transducers is typically called a Capacitance-to-Digital Converter (CDC). A classification of the most common CDC architectures found in the literature is:

- The conversion consists of quantising the period of a relaxation oscillator that is controlled by the capacitance value of the capacitive transducer. The basic block diagram of this type of CDC is presented in Figure 3.16.a. The implementation of a CDC in [60] is based on this architecture. In this design, the capacitive sensor capacitance value (and two other reference capacitors) control the frequency of the relaxation oscillator. In this way, by using a secondary reference clock signal, the number of pulses from the relaxation oscillator are counted. The output of this counter is used on a post-processing algorithm to obtain the capacitance change in the transducer.

- The interface is based on a dual-slope architecture. As shown in Figure 3.16.b, the *first slope* is generated by integrating a known voltage into the capacitor for a fixed amount of time (the slope is variable and depends on the capacitance value). In the second phase, the integrator is discharged with at a fixed slope given by a reference element (the

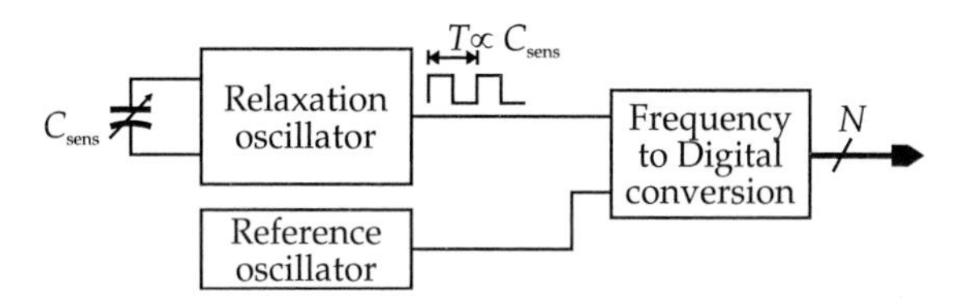

(a) Relaxation oscillator - based CDC

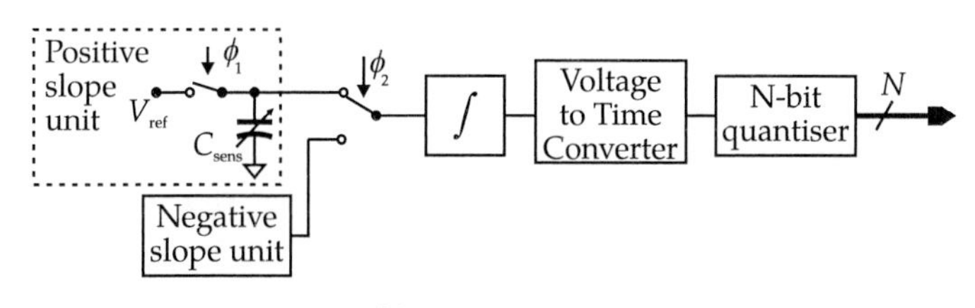

(b) Dual-slope CDC

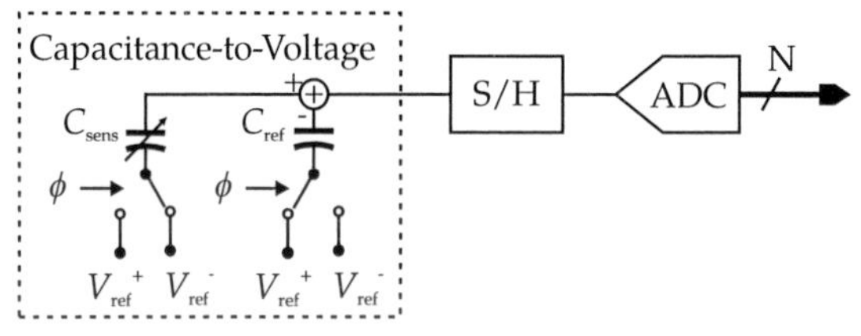

(c) CDC based on CVC and ADC

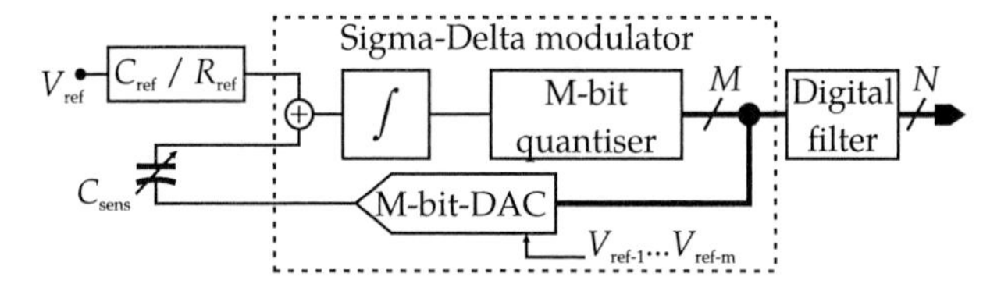

(d) CDC based on a Sigma-Delta modulator

FIGURE 3.16: Simplified block diagrams for common CDC architectures found in the literature.

discharging time is variable). The output of this block represents a Voltage-to-Time Converter (VTC) that then is quantised by a time-to-digital translation. In [61], this type of architecture is implemented by using a capacitor bank as a reference element. On this implementation both slopes are discrete.

- The interface consists of two stages, a Capacitance-to-Voltage Converter (CVC) and an ADC unit as in Figure 3.16.c. In the CVC, the sensing element and a reference capacitor are charged to a known voltage. Through a series of switches and amplifiers, the charge difference of both capacitors is computed and translated into voltage. This voltage is then converted to a digital form using an ADC. The design in [62] is an example of this type of CDC making use of an SAR-ADC.
- The capacitive transducer is located in the loop of a sigma-delta modulator. A generic view of this architecture is presented in Figure 3.16.d. This type of interface provides high-resolution thanks to the use of oversampling. In [63], this architecture is used as an interface by connecting the transducer in a charge-balancing incremental sigma-delta modulator.

The capacitance digitisation method used in the present work is consists of modulating a pulse width base on the measured capacitance (as in a dual-slope architecture). The pulse is the result of comparing the ramps generated by the transducer and a reference capacitor. The conversion is performed by CMOS-Thyristor elements which is a novelty on this kind of converters. In the next paragraphs is presented the architecture proposed, followed by a detailed description of each sub-block.

3.2.2.1 CDC Proposed architecture [64]

Figure 3.17 shows the proposed architecture for the CDC implemented in this work. The capacitive transducer digitisation is done in two stages: first, a Capacitance-to-Time Converter (CTC) is used to generate a pulse whose width is proportional to the capacitance change. This conversion to time is similar to the approach used in the dual-slope CDC. (Figure 3.16.b) for evaluating the slopes (combination of integrator and VTC). The output of the CTC is processed by a Time-to-Digital Converter (TDC) unit. The final output is an N bit digital word corresponding to the change in capacitance that the transducer experienced due to the applied pressure.

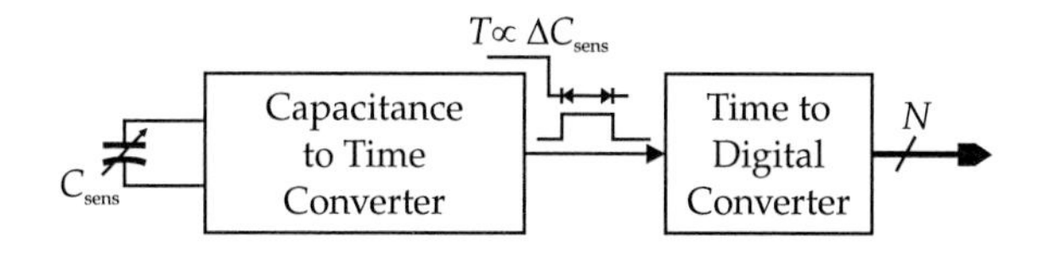

FIGURE 3.17: General view of the architecture proposed for the Capacitance-to-Digital Converter.

A more detailed view of the developed interface is presented in Figure 3.18. The diagram shows the division between the components utilised off-chip and on-chip. To improve the resolution and to reduce the effect of parasitic elements, the measurement is done differentially. Since the capacitive pressure sensor utilised is a two terminals device [65], the use of a secondary reference capacitor (with a fixed value) is necessary. The value of this capacitor is chosen to be equal to offset capacitance C_{offset}, which is the sum of the base capacitance of the sensor and any other mismatch found during the system design phase (e.g. offset strain due to the packaging and the wire-bonds that connect the sensor). If this reference capacitor has a low tolerance, and the PCB and on-chip traces are symmetrical (to equate their contribution on parasitic elements C_{par}), then the CDC sees at its input only the difference in

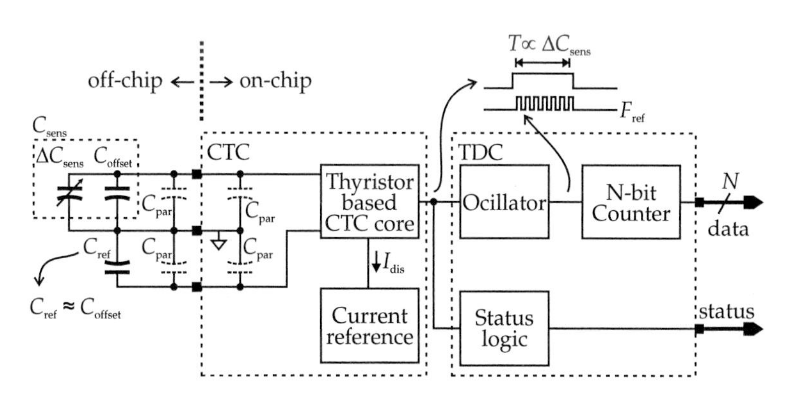

FIGURE 3.18: Detailed block diagram of the implemented CDC, including parasitic capacitor elements.

capacitance due to variations on the effective pressure applied as:

$$\Delta C_{\text{sens}} = C_{\text{sens}} + C_{\text{par}} - (C_{\text{ref}} + C_{\text{par}}) = C_{\text{sens}} - C_{\text{offset}} \,, \tag{3.33}$$

The selection of the reference capacitor and PCB design is a critical task since these offset values and parasitic elements are comparably larger than the capacitance variations due to the pressure (hundreds of femtofarads to single-digit picofarads vs hundreds of attofarads).

The designed CTC is based on the use of CMOS-thyristor circuits as its core element. When this work was written, and to the author knowledge, this is the first time that thyristor circuits are used for a Capacitance-to-Time conversion unit [64]. This core unit is completed with a low-power, Process, Supply Voltage, and Temperature (PVT) independent current source (Figure 3.18). These two blocks allow the CTC to produce a pulse whose width is proportional to the change in capacitance. This pulse is then fed to the TDC to complete the conversion.

The TDC is based on an oscillator and an N-bit counter. As shown in Figure 3.18, the oscillator is restricted to run only during the active time of the pulse generated by the CTC. The clock signal generated has a fixed frequency F_{ref} and is used by the N-bit counter to digitise the duration of the pulse and hence the change in capacitance experienced by the transducer. Also, part of the TDC is a logic for producing some status signals utilised by the implantable device control unit.

3.2.2.2 Capacitance to time conversion [64]

As mentioned early in this chapter, the first stage of the designed interface for digitising the output of the capacitive pressure transducer consists of a conversion of capacitance into a time value. Figure 3.19.a shows a basic block diagram of a CTC, while Figure 3.19.b shows a graph with the most relevant signals involved during the conversion. The control signal V_{rst} defines two phases for the translation. In the first phase ($V_{\text{rst}} = \text{high}$), the capacitor under test (C) is charged to known value V_{ref}. In the second phase ($V_{\text{rst}} = \text{low}$), the capacitor is connected to a constant current source that drains the charge stored on it. This discharge process produces a linear decrease in the capacitor voltage with a slope given by:

$$\frac{\mathrm{d}V}{\mathrm{d}t} = \frac{I_{\text{dis}}}{C} \,, \tag{3.34}$$

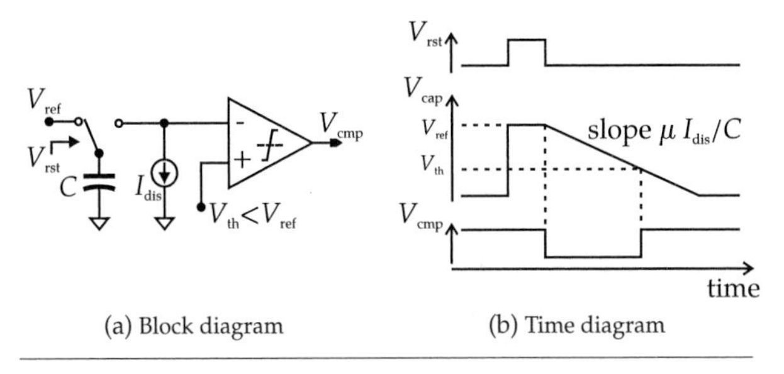

(a) Block diagram (b) Time diagram

FIGURE 3.19: Conceptual diagrams of the process for translating the capacitance value into a pulse width (time).

where I_{dis} is the discharging current. In this case, it is possible to note that for a constant current reference, the slope depends solely on the actual capacitance value. In this way, by comparing the capacitor voltage with a stable threshold, it is possible to produce a pulse whose width is dependent on the capacitance value. For this work, the unit shown in Figure 3.19.a is implemented using a thyristor element.

CMOS Thyristor element

A CMOS Thyristor is formed by a P-MOS and an N-MOS transistor connected in a positive feedback loop. Figure 3.20 presents the circuit diagram of this device. As described in [66], the thyristor is in its *off* state when the tensions at the nodes P_{trig} and N_{trig} are V_{supply} and ground, respectively. At this point, a small leakage current flows through M_{N0} and starts discharging the node P_{trig} to ground (and concurrently the node N_{trig} is charged towards V_{supply} by the leakage current from transistor M_{P0}). At the point when the tension at P_{trig} falls below $V_{supply} - V_{thp}$ (V_{thp} is the threshold voltage of the P-MOS transistor), the positive feedback loop causes the node P_{trig} to quickly discharge to ground (and at the same time a fast charge of the node N_{trig}),

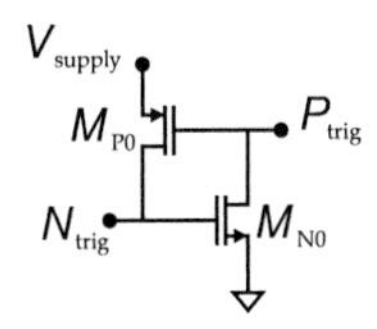

FIGURE 3.20: Basic CMOS thyristor circuit

rushing the system to its *on* state. Power savings are achieved thanks to the lack of direct paths from V_{supply} to ground (except for gate leakage currents), and the rapid transition between states.

Thyristor based CTC core unit

Figure 3.21.a shows the unit cell used for the capacitance to time conversion. This unit, based on [67], adapts the conceptual design presented in Figure 3.20 in such a way that the delay between the *off* and *on* state be dependent on an external capacitor C_{ext}. The capacitor C_{int} is used to balance the large capacitance difference between the nodes N_{trig} and P_{trig} due to the external capacitor. On this unit cell, a trigger signal V_{rst} (and its complementary value $\overline{V_{rst}}$) is used to drive the system to the *off* state. Also, this trigger signal charges the external capacitor C_{ext} to the supply voltage V_{supply} (and discharges C_{int} to ground). Once the signal V_{rst} transitions to its inactive value the transistors M_{P1} and M_{N1} are turn off and the external capacitor (and hence the node P_{trig}) start to discharge towards ground by the reference current I_{dis}. As described previously, this leads to a change of the thyristor state. In this case, and assuming the leakage in M_{N0} is negligible compared to the discharging current source I_{dis}, the time required for the thyristor transition from its *off* to the *on* state is given by [67]:

$$t_d = \frac{C_{ext} V_{thp}}{I_{dis}} + \sqrt[3]{\frac{6C_{ext}^2 C_{int}}{\kappa_p I_{dis}^2}} V_{thn} + \delta t \,, \tag{3.35}$$

where $\kappa_p = \mu_p C_{ox}(W_p/L_p)$, and δt is a regenerative time constant that can be neglected [67]. Since the internal capacitance C_{int}, and the dimensions of the transistors are fixed, and the reference current I_{dis} is constant and PVT independent, the delay time t_d is only a function of the external capacitor.

As described in previous paragraphs, there is a need to perform a differential measurement for the correct reading of the capacitive transducer. This differential measurement allows to cancel noise and to reduce the effects of the parasitic elements shown in Figure 3.18. For this purpose, the differential CTC unit presented in Figure 3.21.b was designed. This module consists of two symmetrical thyristor elements that are synchronised by the positive edge V_{rst} signal, as in Figure 3.21.c. As shown in the Figure 3.21.b, the differential measurement described in Section 3.2.2.1 is achieved by connecting the transducer to one of the thyristors and the reference capacitor to the second one.

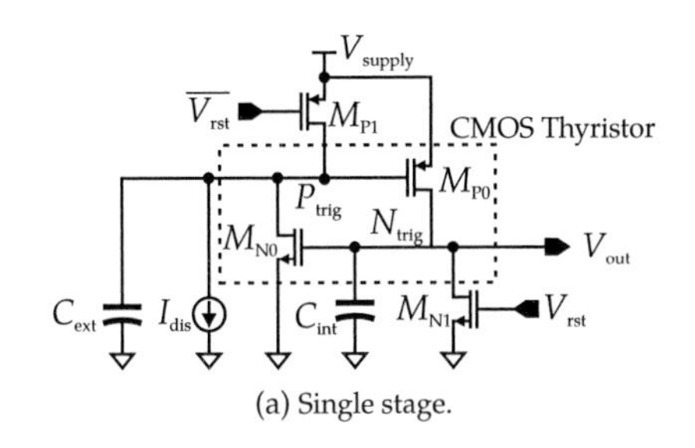

(a) Single stage.

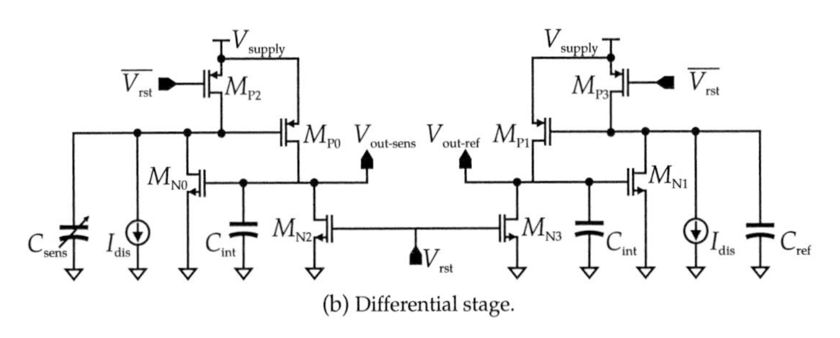

(b) Differential stage.

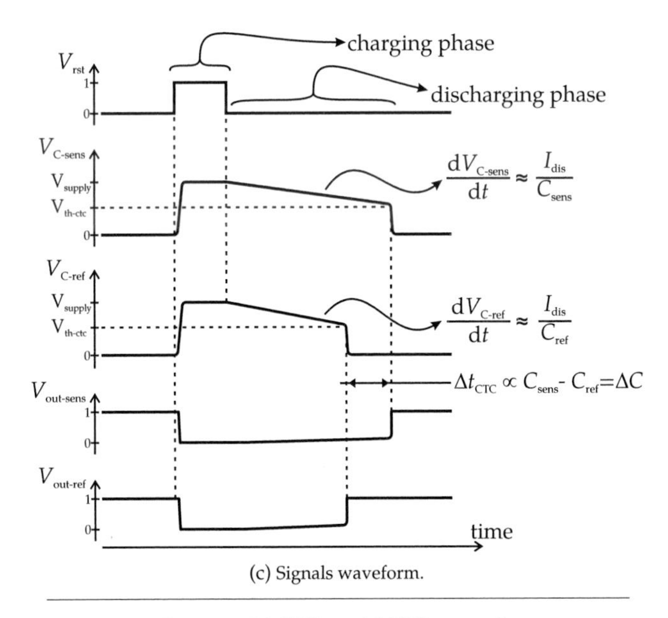

(c) Signals waveform.

FIGURE 3.21: Differential CTC core unit.

Suppose the transducer capacitance is $C_{\text{sens}} = \Delta C + C_{\text{offset}}$ (as in Figure 3.18). In that case, the delay between the negative edge (Figure 3.21.c) of the control signal V_{rst} and the positive edge of the left thyristor element output voltage $V_{\text{out-sens}}$ can be calculated by using Equation 3.35 as:

$$t_{V\text{out-sens}} = \frac{(\Delta C + C_{\text{offset}})V_{\text{thp}}}{I_{\text{dis}}} + \sqrt[3]{\frac{6(\Delta C + C_{\text{offset}})^2 C_{\text{int}}}{\kappa_p I_{\text{dis}}^2}} V_{\text{thn}} + \delta t\,, \quad (3.36)$$

similarly, and by setting $C_{\text{ref}} = C_{\text{offset}}$, the time delay generated on the *reference* thyristor is given by:

$$t_{V\text{out-ref}} = \frac{C_{\text{offset}} V_{\text{thp}}}{I_{\text{dis}}} + \sqrt[3]{\frac{6C_{\text{offset}}^2 C_{\text{int}}}{\kappa_p I_{\text{dis}}^2}} V_{\text{thn}} + \delta t\,, \quad (3.37)$$

since both thyristors in Figure 3.21.b are synchronised by the control signal V_{rst}, the difference between the delays experienced on both branches can be computed by subtracting Equation 3.36 and Equation 3.37:

$$\begin{aligned} \Delta t_{\text{CTC}} &= t_{V\text{out-sens}} - t_{V\text{out-ref}} \\ &= \frac{\Delta C\, V_{\text{thp}}}{I_{\text{dis}}} + \sqrt[3]{\frac{6(\Delta C + C_{\text{offset}})^2 C_{\text{int}}}{\kappa_p I_{\text{dis}}^2}} V_{\text{thn}} \\ &\quad - \sqrt[3]{\frac{6C_{\text{offset}}^2 C_{\text{int}}}{\kappa_p I_{\text{dis}}^2}} V_{\text{thn}} \end{aligned} \quad (3.38)$$

The contribution of the cubic terms in Equation 3.38 is negligible compared to the first term. Given this, the time difference between the positive edges of $V_{\text{out-sens}}$ and $V_{\text{out-ref}}$ (Figure 3.21.c) can be approximated to:

$$\Delta t_{\text{CTC}} \approx \frac{\Delta C\, V_{\text{thp}}}{I_{\text{dis}}} \quad (3.39)$$

The relationship in Equation 3.39 can be used to determine the capacitance change anytime the current reference I_{dis} is stable over the different process and voltage corners. In order to provide a stable I_{dis}, a current reference design can be implemented as described in Appendix A. The symmetry of the current mirrors connected to each branch of the CTC is important to reduce mismatch on the reference currents, which can be reflected as an offset on the capacitance reading.

For completing the interface, a circuit is used to generate a pulse whose

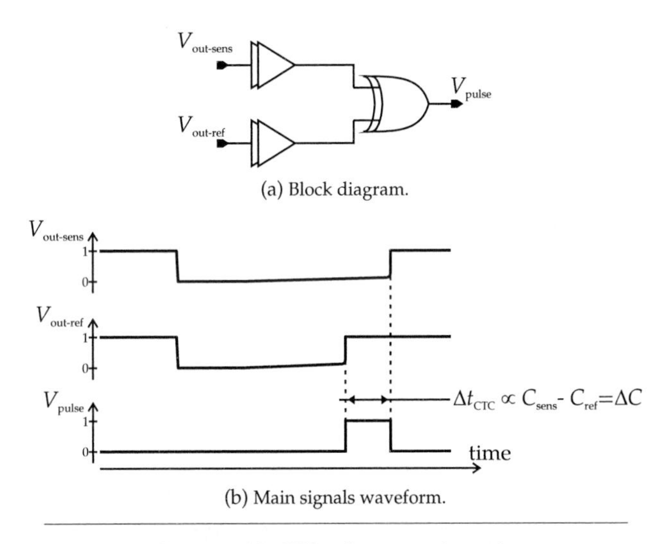

FIGURE 3.22: CTC pulse generation unit.

width is equal to the time difference described by Equation 3.39. The block diagram for the pulse generation unit is shown in Figure 3.22.a. The output of these two paths is processed by an XOR gate that finally produces a pulse whose width is proportional to the transducer capacitance change, as shown in Figure 3.22.b. The symmetry of the two buffer lines, as well the design of the XOR gate, is critical to minimise delay differences between the signals due to any mismatch. In the case of the XOR gate, the use of AOI logic [68] allows for a symmetrical layout that reduces the deviations due to the fabrication process. By taking into account these considerations, the generated pulse corresponds to the output of the thyristor-based CTC as in Equation 3.38.

3.2.2.3 Time to digital conversion [64]

The digital pulse generated in the CTC described in Section 3.2.2.2 has to be converted into a binary word format in order to be processed or stored in a digital system. For this purpose, the Time-to-Digital Converter (TDC) unit shown in Figure 3.23.a is proposed. The concept is based on the use of a relaxation oscillator and an N-bit digital counter. The design of a low-jitter, and PVT invariant relaxation oscillator is critical for the system resolution since any frequency variation results in degradation of the minimum detectable capacitance value.

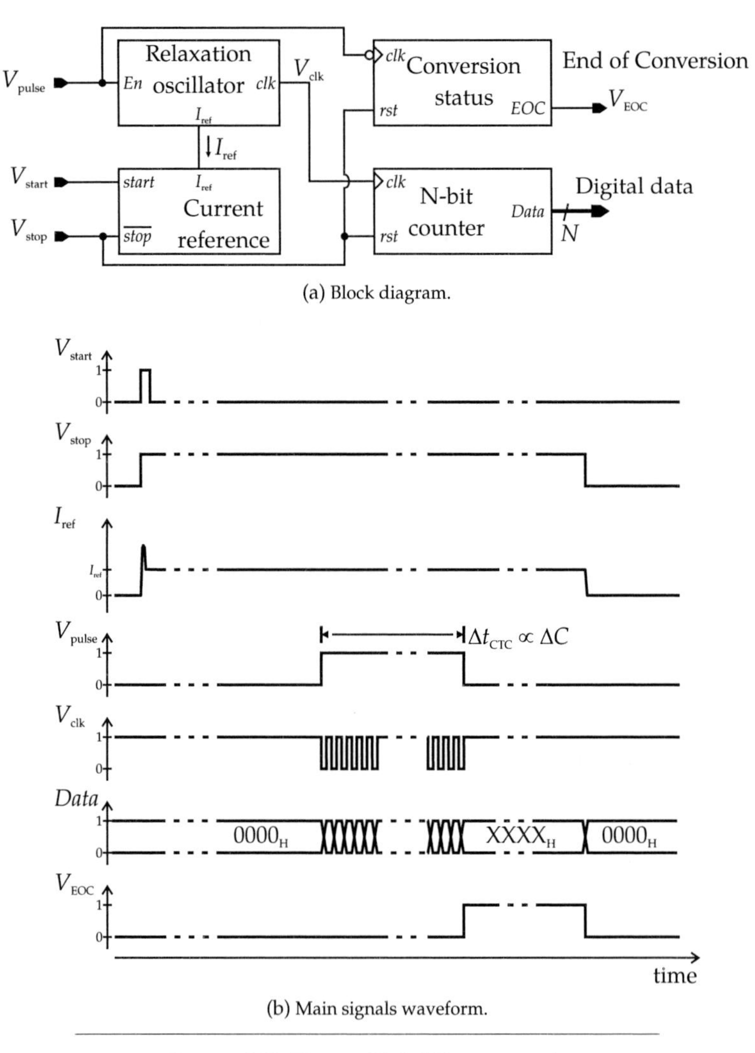

(a) Block diagram.

(b) Main signals waveform.

FIGURE 3.23: Time-to-Digital Converter unit

Relaxation oscillator

Figure 3.24.a presents the circuit diagram of the relaxation oscillator [69]. This design is based on the use of a current-mode comparator and a Schmitt trigger. On both branches of the comparator flows a fixed current I_{ref} which is set by the biasing voltages V_{bias1} and V_{bias2} provided by a current reference circuit as the one described in Appendix A. When the pulse generated in the CTC (Section 3.2.2.2) V_{pulse} is high, the oscillator is enabled through the NAND gate at the output of the Schmitt trigger.

During the pulse V_{pulse}, the current I_{ref} charges the integrating capacitor C_{osc} towards the voltage V_{ref} (produced by the fixed current flowing through

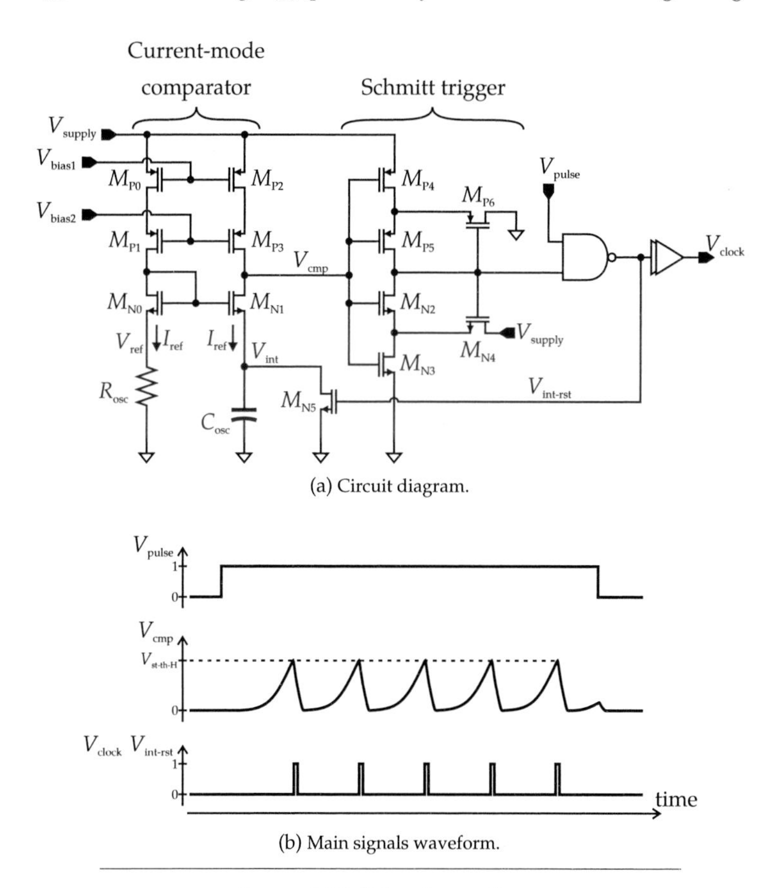

(a) Circuit diagram.

(b) Main signals waveform.

FIGURE 3.24: Relaxation oscillator

R_{osc}). When the voltage in the capacitor V_{int} overpasses V_{ref}, the transistor M_{N1} turns off and then the node voltage V_{cmp} increases rapidly [69]. After a delay, V_{cmp} reaches the highest threshold voltage of the Schmitt trigger section $V_{st-th-H}$ causing a positive pulse in $V_{int-rst}$ (as illustrated in Figure 3.24.b) that turns on the transistor M_{N4} that discharges the integrating capacitor to ground. The reduction in V_{int} makes V_{cmp} also to decrease. The pulse in $V_{int-rst}$ goes back to zero once V_{cmp} falls below the lowest threshold voltage of the Schmitt trigger ($V_{st-th-L}$). This process repeats until the CTC output signal V_{pulse} goes back to low, as shown in Figure 3.24.b. The period of the signal $V_{int-rst}$ can then be calculated as:

$$T_{osc} = R_{osc}C_{osc} + \tau \,, \tag{3.40}$$

where τ is the delay accumulated in the current-mode comparator, the Schmitt trigger and the enable circuit (NAND gate). For keeping this expression valid, it is required to minimise the mismatch between the branches of the current-mode comparator by using appropriate design techniques and good practices. Furthermore, the temperature coefficient of the resistor can also play a role in the frequency stability of this design. For this, [69] proposes to use parallel resistors with complementary temperature coefficients that can cancel each other.

The Schmitt trigger present in the oscillator plays a role in the period of the clock as part of the delay component τ in Equation 3.40. In order to generate the pulses that form the signal $V_{int-rst}$ (and to add noise some immunity to the comparison process), the system exploits the hysteresis of the Schmitt trigger design. As mentioned earlier, V_{cmp} is compared against the threshold voltages of $V_{st-th-H}$ and $V_{st-th-L}$. These threshold voltages can be controlled by the design equations [59]:

$$\frac{\beta_{MN3}}{\beta_{MN4}} = \frac{W_{MN3}L_{MN4}}{L_{MN3}W_{MN4}} = \left[\frac{V_{supply} - V_{st-th-H}}{V_{st-th-H} - V_{thn}}\right]^2 , \tag{3.41}$$

$$\frac{\beta_{MP4}}{\beta_{MP6}} = \frac{W_{MP4}L_{MP6}}{L_{MP4}W_{MP6}} = \left[\frac{V_{st-th-L}}{V_{supply} - V_{st-th-L} - V_{thp}}\right]^2 , \tag{3.42}$$

where W_x and L_x are the width and length of the transistor x.

Digital counter and status logic

The final components of the CTC are the N-bit digital counter and the status logic. In the case of the digital counter, a simple ripple counter is used, since the system does not require high speed, there are no problems with a glitch at the output since it is only evaluated at the end of the conversion. The implementation using the ripple counter optimises the area consumption since it requires less logic gates when compared to a synchronous counter. For the conversion status logic, a negative edge flip flop is used to translate the transition from high to low from the signal V_{pulse} into a level that is detected by the control logic on the implantable device. Both digital blocks are implemented using low power standard cells. Also, the same control signal used to enable the current reference (Appendix A) in the CTC and the relaxation oscillator is utilised as a reset for these digital blocks.

3.2.2.4 Noise analysis on the proposed CDC unit

As with the piezoresistive transducer case, a noise analysis of the capacitive sensor interface allows to get an insight of the noise sources in the device and to take actions at circuit and system level to reduce its effect.

Section 3.2.2.1 described the developed interface and showed that it works in two stages, a capacitance-to-time conversion and a time-to-digital translation. The noise introduction mechanisms depend on the stage characteristics, and therefore each one has a different analysis. The noise sources affecting the capacitance change digitisation are shown in Figure 3.25. The noise analysis is done by following the signal path from the sensing (and reference) capacitors towards the generation of V_{clk} (output).

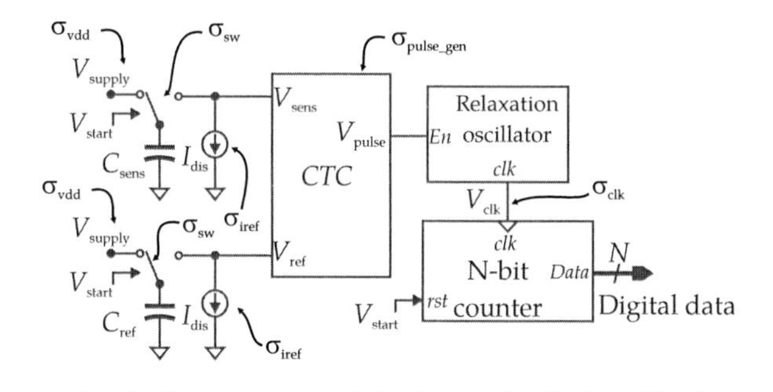

FIGURE 3.25: Noise sources in the CDC unit.

Noise introduced in the CTC.

As described in Section 3.2.2.2, the CTC performs the translation of capacitance into time in two time-separated phases. The noise introduced to the reading has to be studied in each phase to calculate the total uncertainty. Figure 3.20 presented the ideal output of the CTC, where the pulse width of V_{pulse} is proportional to the capacitance difference between the sense and reference capacitors (Equation 3.39). In a real system, the noise present in the system is reflected as a variation on the pulse width, which affects the minimum detectable capacitance change.

Figure 3.26.a shows a graphical representation of the noise effects on either the capacitors C_{sens} and C_{ref} connected to the CTC. The first noise introduction happens during the charging phase, where the capacitor voltage at time t_c (charging time) should ideally be equal to V_{supply}, but in reality, is deviated due to noise. This non-ideal component only shifts the discharging curve in time without changing its slope (as shown in the figure). Additionally, during the discharging phase, the added noise produces a change in the slope of the capacitor voltage curve.

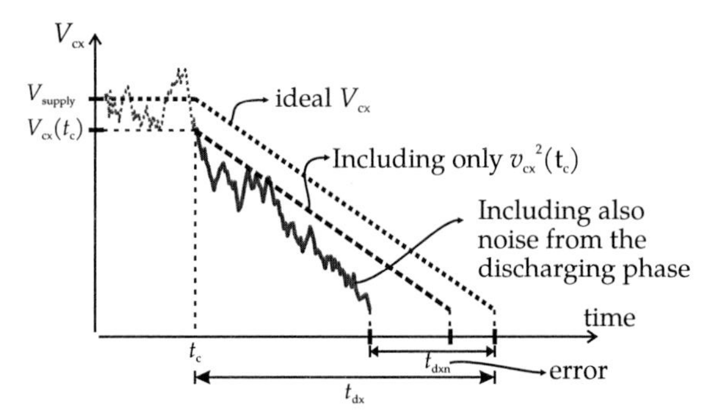

(a) Noise effect on the capacitor voltage when during the capacitance to time conversion.

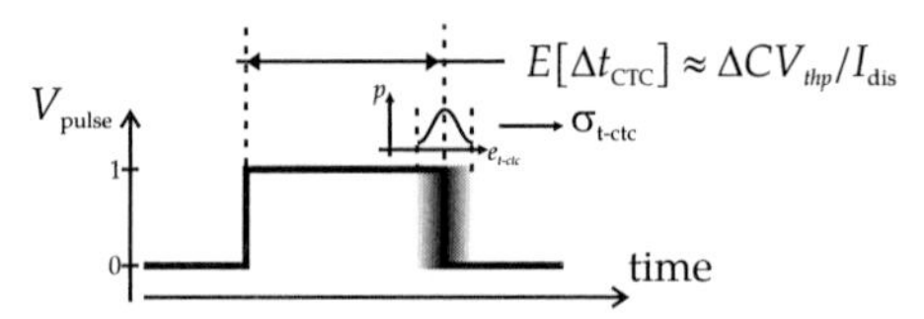

(b) Representation of the error in Δt_{CTC} due to noise.

FIGURE 3.26: Noise effects on the CTC unit (the curves are representative and not to scale).

These random variations on the ideal discharging curves on the sensing and reference capacitors is reflected when generating the output pulse from the CTC, as seen in Figure 3.26.b. Since each capacitor reaches the thyristor threshold earlier or later than expected, the output pulse V_{pulse} width varies in the same way, reducing with it the overall system sensitivity. However, knowing what parameters are related to the pulse width uncertainty $\sigma_{\text{t-ctc}}$ allows designers to mitigate the effect of these noise sources.

As mentioned, the first noise introduction occurs during the charging phase of the sense and reference capacitors. As described in Section 3.2.2.2, during the charging phase, both C_{sens} and C_{ref} are charged towards V_{supply} by using two separate P-MOS matched transistors (M_{P2} and M_{P3} in Figure 3.21.a) as switches. Two noise sources are identified on the charging procedure and are presented in Figure 3.27, the uncertainty of the supply voltage $v_{\text{n,vdd,tc}}$ at time t_{c}, and kT/C noise due to the thermal noise on the finite switch resistance [59]. Flicker noise is neglected since the capacitor is fully charged, and there is no DC current flowing through it [59]. By adding these two noise sources, and assuming that the charging time is larger than the system time constant during this phase, the uncertainty of the capacitor voltage at t_{c} is given by

$$v_{\text{n,c}x}(t_{\text{c}})^2 = v_{\text{n,vdd,tc}}^2 + v_{\text{ktc}x\text{,tc}}^2 \,. \tag{3.43}$$

During the second phase, both capacitors are disconnected from the supply rail, and the discharging process is triggered. In this phase, the pre-charged (ideally to the supply voltage) capacitor is discharged at a constant rate by a fixed current source I_{dis}. The conversion of capacitance is done by detecting when the voltage in the capacitor reaches the thyristor switching threshold (V_{thp} of M_{P1} in Figure 3.21.a). The noise affects the detection and therefore an estimation error of the *discharging time* $t_{\text{d}x}$ occurs (as shown in Figure 3.26.a).

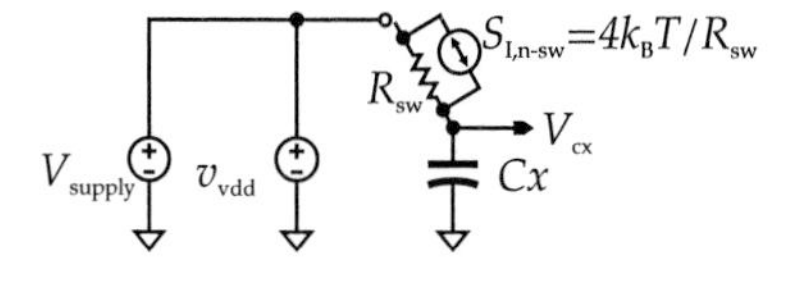

FIGURE 3.27: Noise sources and their relationship during the charging phase in the CTC unit.

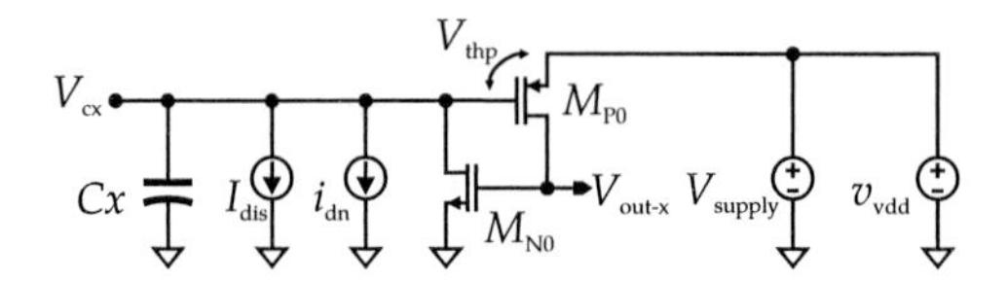

FIGURE 3.28: Noise sources and their relationship during the discharging phase in the CTC unit.

The noise sources during this phase are presented in the simplified diagram in Figure 3.28. In this analysis, two noise sources are identified to be leading to errors on the estimation of the discharging time t_{dx}. The first one is the noise in the current reference circuitry, which affects the discharging slope. The second error component is produced by the noise in the supply source since it affects the switching point of the thyristor.

During the discharging phase, the voltage in the capacitor decays with a nominal slope I_{dis}/C_x, and after a discharging time t_{dx} its value is equal to [70, 71]:

$$V_{cx}(t_{dx}) + v_{n,cx}(t_{dx}) = V_{cx}(t_c) - \frac{1}{C_x}\left(\int_0^{t_{dx}} I_{dis}\,dt + \int_0^{t_{dx}} i_{n,dis}\,dt\right), \quad (3.44)$$

where $i_{n,dis}$ is the noise component from the current reference circuit (Figure 3.28), $v_{n,cx}$ is the total noise in the capacitor voltage, and $V_{cx}(t_c)$ is the capacitor voltage at the end of the charging phase (including noise $v_{n,cx}(t_c)$). The noise $i_{n,dis}$ is uniformly distributed, and its integration into voltage is a Wiener process [70]. The previous means, that the noise component integrated into the capacitor from $i_{n,dis}$ represents a random walk which is a non-stationary process with zero average (around the ideal discharging curve) and a variance that increases with time as represented in Figure 3.29.

Given the characteristics of the noise voltage generated by $i_{n,dis}$, the calculation of the discharging time uncertainty $t^2_{n,i,dx}$ is influenced by two factors: The expected value of the time required to reach the thyristor threshold $E[t_{dx}] = C_x V_{thp}/I_{dis}$ (dominant term in Equation 3.35) and the average voltage slope at the crossing point as in Equation 3.34. In this way (and based on the analysis from [72]), the variance of the discharging time t_{dx},

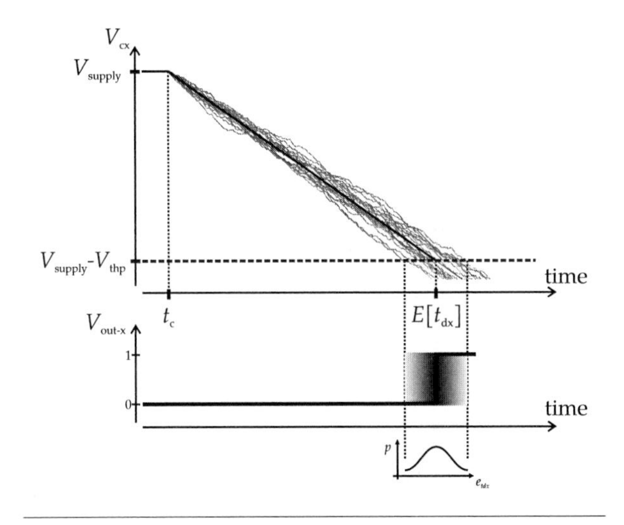

FIGURE 3.29: Noise sources and their relationship during the discharging phase in the CTC unit.

including the effect of the supply line noise, is calculated as:

$$t^2_{\mathrm{n,i,d}x} = \frac{S_{\mathrm{n,idis}} t_{\mathrm{d}x}}{2I^2_{\mathrm{dis}}} + \frac{v^2_{\mathrm{n,vdd,td}x} C^2_x}{I^2_{\mathrm{dis}}} = \frac{C_x}{I^2_{\mathrm{dis}}} \left(\frac{S_{\mathrm{n,idis}} V_{\mathrm{thp}}}{2I_{\mathrm{dis}}} + v^2_{\mathrm{n,vdd,td}x} C_x \right) , \quad (3.45)$$

where $S_{\mathrm{n,idis}}$ is the one-sided Power Spectral Density (PSD) of the noise source $i_{\mathrm{n,dis}}$ (if a two-sided PSD is used, then the first term denominator does not contains the factor 2 [72, 73]), and $v_{\mathrm{n,vdd,td}x}$ is the error on the power supply node at time $t_{\mathrm{d}x}$. This equation makes evident the relationship between the discharging time, which is proportional to the total capacitance (C_x includes parasitic elements), and the magnitude of the effect of the noise in the final reading. The current PSD expression depends on the implemented current reference and mirrors [74].

The error component, introduced in $t_{\mathrm{d}x}$, due to the noise sampled during the charging phase is calculated by dividing the voltage noise components from Equation 3.43 by the average slope [72]:

$$t^2_{\mathrm{n,v,c}x} = \frac{v^2_{\mathrm{n,vdd,tc}} C^2_x}{I^2_{\mathrm{dis}}} + \frac{k_{\mathrm{B}} T C_x}{I^2_{\mathrm{dis}}} , \quad (3.46)$$

By assuming an ideal pulse generation circuit (Figure 3.22.a), based on Equation 3.39, the pulse width uncertainty $t^2_{\mathrm{n,ctc-1}}$ can be calculated by computing and adding the error sources (Equations 3.45 and 3.46) introduced on the sensor and reference branches of the CTC:

$$\begin{aligned} t^2_{\mathrm{n,ctc-1}} &= t^2_{\mathrm{n,csens}} + t^2_{\mathrm{n,cref}} = t^2_{\mathrm{n,i,d-sens}} + t^2_{\mathrm{n,v,c-sens}} + t^2_{\mathrm{n,i,d-ref}} + t^2_{\mathrm{n,v,c-ref}} \\ &= \left(\frac{S_{\mathrm{n,idis}} V_{\mathrm{thp}}}{2 I^3_{\mathrm{dis}}} + \frac{k_B T}{I^2_{\mathrm{dis}}} \right) (C'_{\mathrm{sens}} + C'_{\mathrm{ref}}) \, , \\ &\quad + \frac{v^2_{\mathrm{n,vdd,tdx}}}{I^2_{\mathrm{dis}}} (C'^2_{\mathrm{sens}} + C'^2_{\mathrm{ref}}) \end{aligned} \tag{3.47}$$

where C'_{sens} and C'_{ref} also include the total parasitic capacitance on the sense and reference CTC inputs, respectively. It is also important to note that the components from the supply voltage from the charging phase (Equation 3.46) are common for both branches in Figure 3.22.a and therefore get cancelled.

In the case of the pulse generator, the delay lines (implemented as a set of N buffers in series) and the XOR gate also introduce some error to the pulse width. For the minimum design, the delay is formed by two inverters in series per branch and an AOI-logic-based XOR gate. By following a similar procedure as with the rest of the CTC and [72, 75], and assuming perfect matching with same device sizing on each logic gate, the total error introduced in the pulse generation stage can be approximated to:

$$\begin{aligned} t^2_{\mathrm{n,ctc-2}} &= \frac{24 k_B T C_g t_{\mathrm{pd}}}{I_{\mathrm{sat}} V_{\mathrm{supply}}} \left(1 + \frac{4 V_{\mathrm{supply}}}{3(V_{\mathrm{supply}} - V_{\mathrm{th}})} \right) \\ &\quad + 6 t^2_{\mathrm{pd}} \left[\frac{(\alpha - 1) V_{\mathrm{supply}} + V_{\mathrm{th}}}{V_{\mathrm{supply}} - V_{\mathrm{th}}} \right]^2 \left(\frac{\sigma^2_{\mathrm{supply}}}{V^2_{\mathrm{supply}}} \right) \\ &= \frac{6 k_B T C_g}{I^2_{\mathrm{sat}}} \left(1 + \frac{4 V_{\mathrm{supply}}}{3(V_{\mathrm{supply}} - V_{\mathrm{th}})} \right) \\ &\quad + 6 \left[\frac{(\alpha - 1) V_{\mathrm{supply}} + V_{\mathrm{th}}}{V_{\mathrm{supply}} - V_{\mathrm{th}}} \right]^2 \left(\frac{\sigma^2_{\mathrm{supply}} C^2_g}{4 I^2_{\mathrm{sat}}} \right) , \end{aligned} \tag{3.48}$$

where C_g is the input capacitance of the logic gates used, t_{pd} is the average input-to-output propagation delay on each gate, α is the velocity saturation index (from the alpha-power model [72, 76]), and I_{sat} is the saturation current calculated as $(1/2)\mu C_{\mathrm{ox}}(W/L)(V_{\mathrm{supply}} - V_{\mathrm{th}})^2$.

Together Equations 3.47 and 3.48 describe the total uncertainty introduced in the proposed CTC unit. In the case of the pulse generation sub-block, it is relevant to note that choosing logic gates with minimum propagation delay (t_{pd}) reduces the overall error introduced during this stage (Equation 3.48). The impact of using fast logic gates for the implementation of this block is reduced since each gate transitions only two times during the whole conversion process keeping the dynamic power contribution minimum. Furthermore, from Equation 3.47, it is clear the impact that parasitic and offset capacitance has on the error. Finally, Equation 3.45 provides a design criterion for the discharging current. Larger values on I_{dis} leads to reduction of the uncertainty in the capacitance to time conversion stage but at the price of a direct increase on the power consumption of the CTC. Also, and indirectly, the TDC power consumption is proportional to I_{dis} since it reduces the conversion time, meaning that a faster clock is required to keep the same capacitance resolution.

Noise introduced in the TDC.

The TDC unit presented in Section 3.2.2.3 consists of an oscillator and a counter. In this unit, two noise sources are present: electric noise introduced in the oscillator that causes jitter, and the time digitisation process adds quantisation noise.

The period variations in the oscillator unit, known as jitter, are reflected as noise in the pulse width estimation. The jitter calculation depends on the type of oscillator implemented. As presented in Section 3.2.2.3, the current design implements a relaxation oscillator for generating the clock signal. As shown in the waveforms from Figure 3.24.b, the oscillator is based on the charge and discharge of a capacitor. This process resembles that explained for the thyristor-based CTC; consequently, a similar error introduction mechanism is expected: The noise in the charging current source (I_{ref} in Figure 3.24.a) is integrated in the capacitor C_{osc}, this is reflected on the comparison causing variations on the switching time. These variations are hence reflected as jitter. Following a similar approach as for the thyristor-based CTC, the jitter produced in the oscillator can be approximated to [77]:

$$t_{n,osc}^2 = \frac{2k_B T}{I_{ref}^2 R_{osc} f_{osc}} + \frac{S_{n,iref}}{2I_{ref}^2 f_{osc}}, \tag{3.49}$$

where $S_{n,iref}$ is the one-sided PSD of the current reference noise, and f_{osc} is the oscillator's nominal frequency. There is also some additional jitter added by the smith trigger block and buffers, yet it can be neglected since the slopes are fast [77].

Previously it was also indicated that there is quantisation noise added during the time digital estimation. Given that each quantisation step is equal to a single period from the clock generator T_{osc}, the noise introduced during the final digitisation stage is given by [52]:

$$\sigma^2_{\text{qCDC}} = \frac{T^2_{\text{osc}}}{12} \,. \tag{3.50}$$

The results from Equations 3.47, 3.48, 3.49 and 3.50 provide designers with a description of the noise in this novel interface based on thyristors. With these equations, it is possible to define a noise budget expression that can be used together with the design specifications to define the interface parameters properly.

The next section presents the experimental results for the described interface after being implemented in a test ASIC. Some of the results are used to validate the expressions previously described.

3.2.2.5 CDC implementation and results [64]

The novel concept for the thyristor-based Capacitance-to-Digital Converter (CDC) was implemented and fabricated in a 350 nm CMOS process (as part of the test ASIC shown in Section B.1). Figure 3.30 shows an annotated micrograph of the implemented CDC. The total area of the unit is 0.055 mm^2, from which the CTC only occupies 0.03 mm^2.

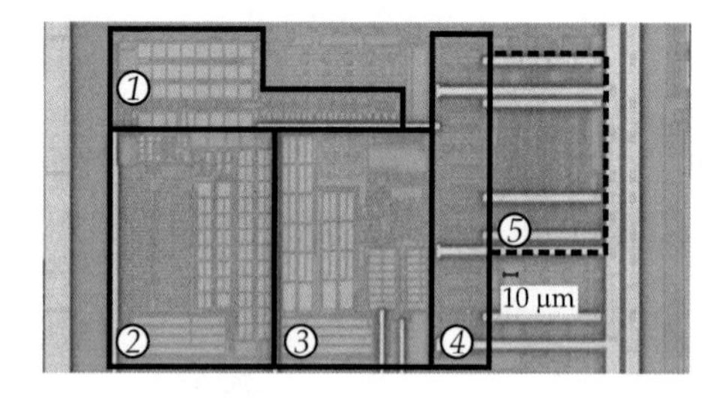

FIGURE 3.30: Annotated micrograph of the CDC implemented in 350 nm CMOS technology. 1. Capacitance-to-Time Converter, 2. CTC Current reference, 3. Relaxation oscillator (clock generation), 4. Ripple counter, 5. SPI interface (test only).

In the next paragraphs, the results from the implemented design are introduced. First, the test setup considerations are described. Then the relaxation oscillator results are presented so that its error magnitude can be known. In the third part of this section, the CDC results and their uncertainty are shown and analysed. Finally, the power consumption and final thoughts on the CDC interface implementation are presented.

Test setup

Ten sample ICs were packaged in a QFN64 package. For test purposes the following signals were accessible from the ASIC pads (and package pins):

TABLE 3.1: Pin-out for the implemented CDC unit

Signal/pad	Direction	Description
CDC_VDD	Input	This is the supply input for the module.
CDC_SENS	Input	Capacitive sensor input (positive node).
CDC_REF	Input	Reference capacitor input (positive node).
CDC_START	Input	*Start* measurement signal.
CDC_STOP	Input	*Stop* module signal.
CDC_EOC	Output	End-of-conversion output.
CDC_PULSE	Output	Test node for the CTC *pulse* output.
CDC_CLK	Output	Test node for the CDC *clock* output.
CDC_EN_TEST	Input	Enable test-mode. Controls the test mode pads. The test-mode drains extra 35 µA.
CDC_CS	Input	SPI interface Chip select input.
CDC_SCLK	Input	SPI Serial clock input.
CDC_SDA	Output	SPI Serial data output (MSB first).

It is necessary to indicate that a simplified SPI interface was included in the implemented design (not indicated in Figure 3.30) to reduce the number of pins required. This interface is connected to the 16 bits parallel output of the CDC, and it loads its value with the positive edge of the end-of-conversion signal. As shown in Table 3.1, the CTC output (*pulse* in Figure 3.22) and the relaxation oscillator clock signal ($V_c lock$ in Figure 3.24) can be monitored in a *test*-mode which is enabled through the pad CDC_EN_TEST.

As part of the test setup, a capacitive transducer had to be selected. In the case of the current work, a commercially available device [78] was chosen. A picture of this sensing element is shown in Figure 3.31. This absolute pressure sensor is formed by an array of 16 membranes fabricated in polysilicon (visible in Figure 3.31), following a similar design as in [65]. Furthermore, fused silica

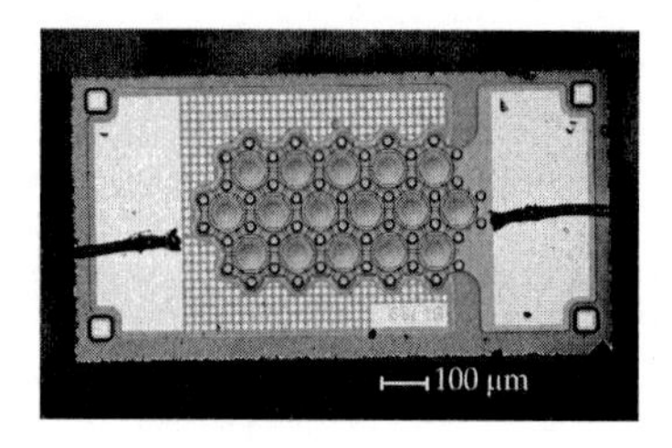

FIGURE 3.31: Capacitive sensor used during the characterisation of the CDC (top view).

was used as a substrate for this transducer, which ensures that this is a floating device with reduced parasitic capacitance.

In order to provide a platform for testing the CDC, the board shown in Figure 3.32 was designed and assembled. The board includes the previously described capacitive sensor, a micro-controller, a low noise LDO regulator and a socket for QFN-64 packaged ICs. The test board was also provided with a footprint to directly wire-bond a bare die of the ASIC.

For the measurement of the timing (e.g. relaxation oscillator frequency) and electrical characteristics of the CDC unit, a test setup consisting of the board in Figure 3.32, a low noise power source, an oscilloscope with data logging function and a sub-femtoampere meter (for current measurement), were used. In these measurements, the micro-controller in the platform board was programmed to perform automatically several measurement cycles with a fixed sampling time. Also, the firmware included the option of disabling the *test-mode* and the SPI interface reading. The later is useful for calculating the power consumption of only the CDC unit and its different components.

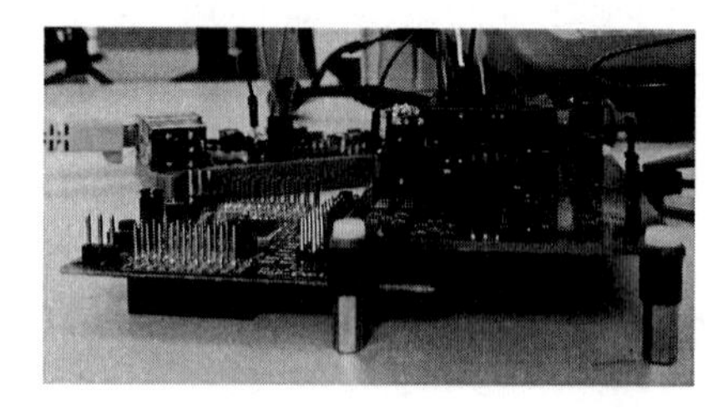

FIGURE 3.32: Test board used for characterising the CDC unit.

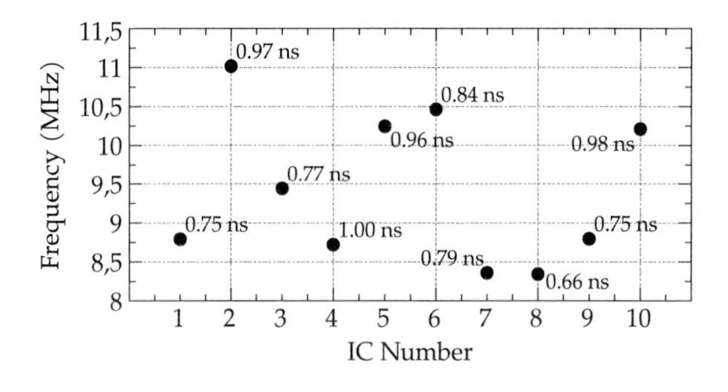

FIGURE 3.33: Average frequency and RMS jitter measured at the output of the relaxation oscillator for the ten sample ICs.

For the tests related to pressure measurement, the controlled pressure and temperature chamber described in Appendix C was adapted and used. The code of the microcontroller in the platform board (Figure 3.32) was modified to keep the *test-mode* disabled all the time and to take samples only when receiving a command from an external reading unit. Furthermore, the automated data logging interface in the test chamber was modified to communicate with the board microcontroller and to process the 16 bits of data coming from the CDC. As described in Appendix C, the logged data is stored in a CSV file for further processing.

Relaxation oscillator results

The first module to verify was the clock generation unit whose core is the relaxation oscillator presented in Section 3.2.2.3. For this test, the system was placed in *test-mode* so that the clock output was fed to the CDC_CLK pad. A high speed oscilloscope with a data logger function was used to save several clock periods while the CDC performed its measurement cycle. The result for the ten sample ICs is shown in Figure 3.33. From these results, the average frequency for the clock is 9.44 MHz, with a standard deviation of 0.9714 MHz.

The RMS jitter was extracted from the CTC clock measurements, and as displayed in Figure 3.33, it does not exceed 1.00 ns. Based on the approximation in Equation 3.39 and nominal parameters, this maximum jitter translates into an error in the capacitance measurement of 1.33 aF, which is negligible compared to the sensitivity of the transducer [78]. The implementation of this unit was dimensioned to get a large margin that accounts for variations and uncertainties of the thyristor-based CTC, the transducer sensitivity and offset, as well as leakage currents. The value of jitter obtained allows to characterise the novel thyristor-based CTC with a minimum distortion from the clock used in the TDC unit.

CDC results

As mentioned in this section, the chamber from Appendix C was adapted to perform the measurements for the CDC unit. By using this setup, steps of 50 mmHg in the range 800 mmHg to 950 mmHg were applied to the system for each sample IC, while keeping the temperature at 37 °C. The resulting curves are shown in Figure 3.34. From this figure, it is possible to note the distribution of the offset between the different tested ICs as well as the linear behaviour in the pressure region.

In a second verification stage, the same test was performed for different temperatures in the range 30 °C to 42 °C. These results, together with the data from the previous test, are summarised in Table 3.2. As presented in the table, the spread of the slopes on each tested IC is small with a deviation $\sigma_{slope\_cdc} = 3.99\ \mathrm{mmHg}^{-1}$.

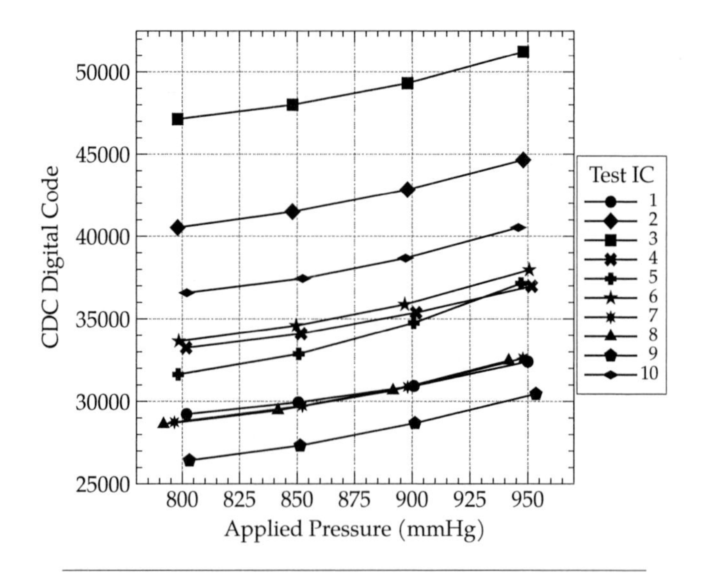

FIGURE 3.34: CDC digital output code versus applied pressure (steps of 50 mmHg at 37 °C).

TABLE 3.2: Average slope, offset and offset drift for each sample IC.

IC	T = 37 °C		T = 37 °C to 42 °C
	Slope ($mmHg^{-1}$)	**Offset***	**Absolute Offset drift (°C^{-1})**
1	21.26	12012.35	50.70
2	27.42	18446.08	123.10
3	27.17	25205.46	122.47
4	24.93	13068.67	16.32
5	36.95	1805.86	5.57
6	28.35	10747.44	13.32
7	25.40	8299.87	18.95
8	25.47	8229.42	32.24
9	26.87	4655.35	28.02
10	27.44	14317.04	61.78

* Extrapolated to 0 mmHg.

The measured gain or slope drift with respect of temperature was found to be negligible ($< 10^{-15}\,°C^{-1}$). In the other hand, the offset presents a much larger dispersion of $\sigma_{offset\_cdc} = 6739.24\,°C^{-1}$. Moreover, in the case of the offset, its drift due to the temperature change represents a more significant parameter. The average offset drift was found to be 47.25 $°C^{-1}$. However, system calibration can solve this problem so that the effect of this drift can be cancelled in post-processing.

The minimum detectable change in capacitance achieved by the interface depends on the total noise present on it. From the previous section, Equations 3.47, 3.48, 3.49 and 3.50 describe the noise introduced in each stage of the developed CDC unit. For these expressions, it is required to take into account that the implemented CDC uses cascode current mirrors biased in the sub-threshold region. In this way, the expression for the current noise PSD in Equations 3.47 and 3.49 is given by $S_{n,i} = 2k_B T g_m$ [79]. Furthermore, the test setup used a low power LDO with a nominal RMS output noise of 30 µV. Under these conditions, the theoretical uncertainty expected in the interface is about 861.92 ns or 8.14 LSB (based on the average clock of 9.44 MHz from the oscillator's results).

The design margin for the TDC is evident when computing the theoretical error values: The total error introduced in the TDC (i.e. oscillator jitter and quantisation noise) is $\sigma^2_{TDC} = 836.38 \times 10^{-18}\,s^2$, while for the CTC it is

$\sigma^2_{\text{CTC}} = 742.07 \times 10^{-15}\,\text{s}^2$. This considerable difference between these error contributions attenuates the effect of design or noise deviations, at the TDC, over the overall results. In this way, a better characterisation of the novel thyristor-based CDC can be done. However, the next paragraphs reveal that this is done at the expense of increased power consumption by the TDC.

A modified version of the test board in Figure 3.32 was fabricated to validate the previous results. In this board, the capacitive transducer and the reference capacitor were both replaced by fixed elements of (6.50 ± 0.05) pF. This modification was done with the purpose to remove the dependency on the pressure and then provide a theoretical $\Delta C = 0\ F$. In this way, the maximum uncertainty between measurement cycles can be extracted. For this test, the supply voltage was set to 3.3 V, and the temperature was set to 37 °C. Also, as part of the test setup, the microcontroller was configured to instruct the CDC to perform a new measurement cycle every 50 ms (sampling frequency of 20 Hz).

With the previously described setup, a long-term (about 50 s to get 1000 samples) test was performed for each of the sample ICs resulting in the data presented in Figure 3.35. The data collected during this test results in an average uncertainty of 818 ns or 8.2 LSB. The obtained values are consistent with the theory presented in the previous paragraph. Validating in this way the noise analysis described in Section 3.2.2.4.

This measured uncertainty values indicate that the minimum observable

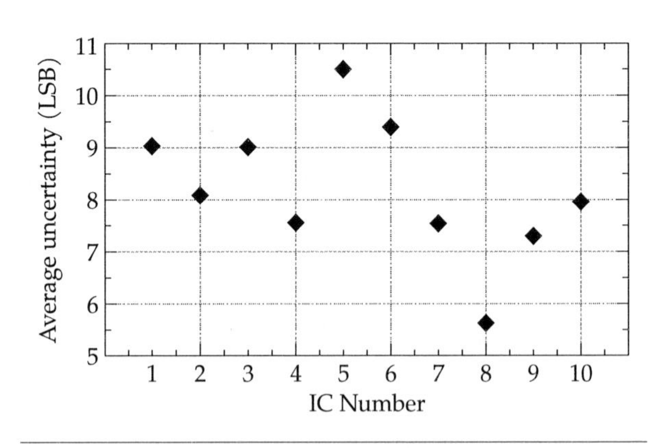

FIGURE 3.35: Average uncertainty in LSB measured for each sample ICs.

change in capacitance is 102 aF, which then translates to a pressure resolution of 0.3 mmHg (based on the selected transducer [78]). This uncertainty lies mainly on the CTC pulse generation deviations and jitter from the clock in the TDC. The capacitance resolution obtained allows then to calculate that the interface ENOB [61] is 12.95.

A verification of the previous results was done by using the modified pressure chamber together with the capacitive transducer [78]. The results are limited to the minimum achievable pressure steps in the test setup, which was 0.5 mmHg. The described test was performed over the sample IC number 5 (presenting the higher uncertainty in Figure 3.35), for the pressure range 850 mmHg to 856 mmHg and at a fixed temperature of 37 °C. The results of this test are shown in Figure 3.36.a. A best-fit INL analysis was performed for the tested points to provide information of the deviations in the interface. As seen in Figure 3.36.b, the error is around the expected uncertainty for the tested IC (Figure 3.35) and therefore represents an acceptable error level.

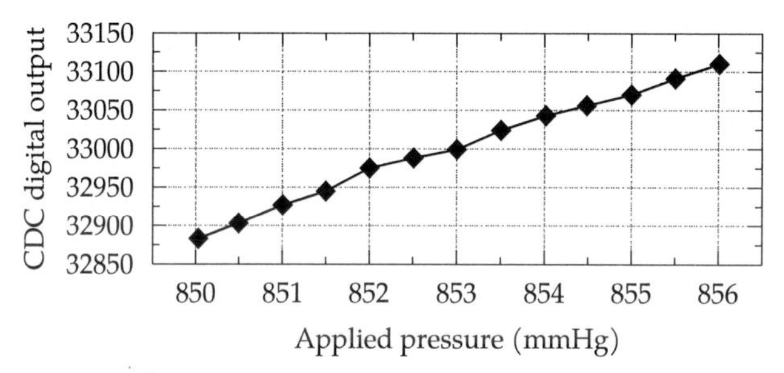

(a) CDC digital output code versus applied pressure.

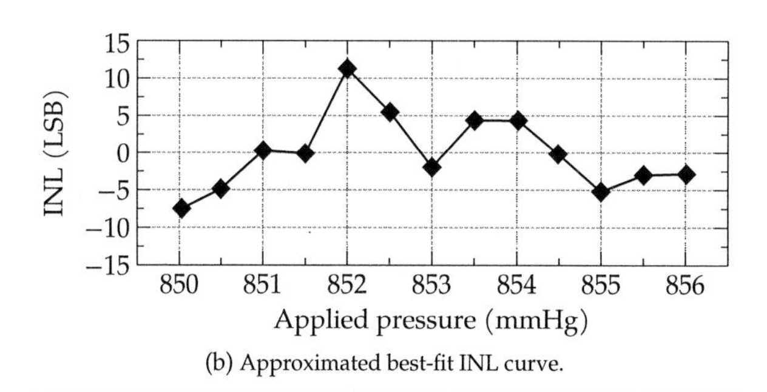

(b) Approximated best-fit INL curve.

FIGURE 3.36: CDC response under minimum pressure changes (steps of 0.5 mmHg at 37 °C, sample IC number 5).

Power consumption of the implemented CDC unit

Given that this unit is intended for use in miniaturised IMS, its power consumption is a critical parameter. As described in Appendix 3.2.2.2, the use of CMOS thyristors for the conversion of capacitance to time provides power savings by limiting the amount of current flowing to ground. In order to interpret the results for power measurement of the interface, it is essential to define the current profile of the system during operation. Figure 3.37.a shows an oscilloscope capture of the power profile of one of the sample ICs when a capacitance conversion is being performed. Short transient peaks occur during the transition of operation phases. Moreover, a large spike appears at the startup of the current references (i.e., at the edges of the V_{start} signal, Appendix A). However, these spikes are limited on time and can be neglected from the system average power consumption.

The different phases in the power profile are described in Figure 3.37.b. By the application of a high level to V_{stop} and a short pulse in V_{start}, the system charges the sensing and reference capacitors. This charging action and the triggering of the current references produces, as mentioned earlier, a transient consumption peak. However, once V_{start} is released, the power consumption remains low with only the CTC active (darker area in Figure 3.37.b). This level energy is dominant for most of the operation time of the CDC. In this phase, the capacitors are discharging at a constant rate, and the energy is consumed mainly by the current reference circuit and a small amount used by the CTC thyristor circuits. Once the output V_{pulse} (from the CTC) goes high, the actual conversion of ΔC begins (Appendix 3.2.2.3). In this region, the power consumption is maximum since the oscillator, and digital circuitry becomes active.

As presented in Figure 3.37.b, the time each phase is active depends on the effective values (nominal capacitance and parasitics) of the sensing ($C_{\text{sens}_{\text{e}}\text{ff}}$) and reference ($C_{\text{sens}_{\text{e}}\text{ff}}$) capacitors. As shown, the total capacitance to digital conversion depends on the maximum capacitance value seen at the sense or reference input nodes. In contrast, the time to digital conversion phase depends on the actual capacitance difference between the capacitive transducer and the reference capacitor. Therefore the total energy consumption of the interface is not fixed for all possible inputs but depends on their actual value. This characteristic can be used at the system design level to optimise the power consumption. Reducing the parasitic and offset values on both the transducer and reference element leads to power savings mainly on the CTC unit. Furthermore, limiting the pressure range, and hence the ΔC, as well as choosing the right value for the reference capacitor, reduces the power consumption during conversion, which provides the significant energy savings for the interface.

Due to the power profile variation based on the input values, the characterisation of the interface was done for the worst-case scenario, which is when a full range conversion is performed. Under this condition, the ten ICs were tested, and their power consumption measured. It was determined that the average power usage for the CTC is 2.99 µW, while when including the TDC, the total average power consumption increases to 20.83 µW.

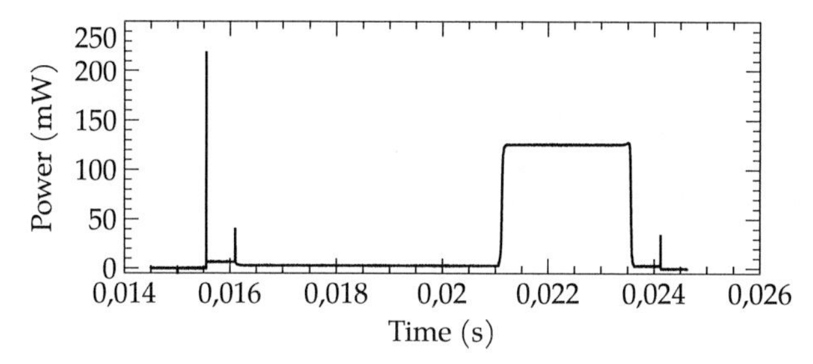

(a) Measured power profile.

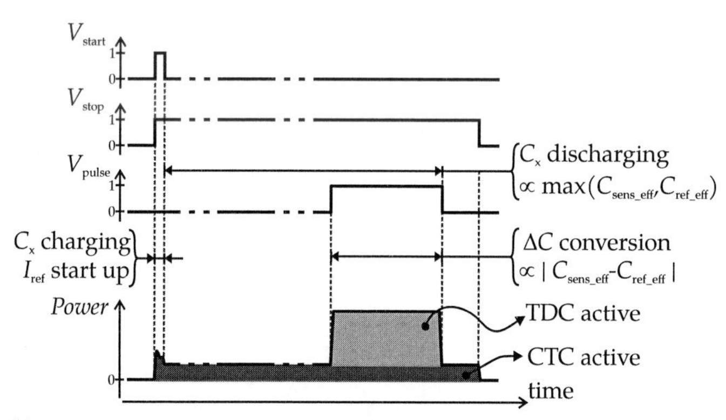

(b) Contributions to the power consumption (representative diagram, not to scale).

FIGURE 3.37: Power profile during CDC operation.

Summary of the CDC interface results

Table 3.3 shows the most important results for the implemented interface for capacitive pressure sensors. The novel use of thyristors for the capacitance to time conversion shows promising results in area and power consumption. The TDC unit has a flexible architecture that can be adapted to reduce the power consumption further as well area utilisation. By adjusting the unit to the requirements of a specific IMS, it is possible to fulfil restrictive power budgets.

TABLE 3.3: Summary results for the implemented CDC unit.

	Thyristor-based CTC	Full interface
Area (mm^2)	0.03	0.055
Supply (V)	2.7 - 3.3	
Active power (μW)	2.99	20.83
Conversion time (ms)	11.1	
Capacitance resolution (aF)	102	
Pressure resolution (mmHg)	0.3	
ENOB (bits)	12.95	
FoM (pJ/conv)	4.19	29.22

Chapter 4

Temperature Monitoring

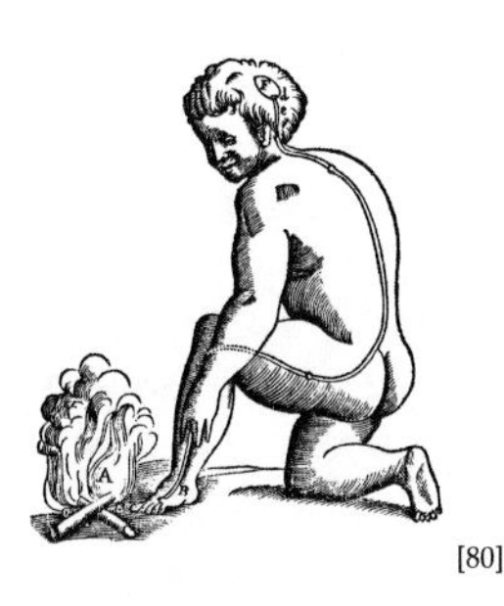

[80]

In physics, the average molecular kinetic energy in a substance is known as temperature. This physical quantity is an essential parameter for living beings. Any small change in temperature influence greatly the metabolisms of living organisms. Extreme temperatures can be threatening for life, too elevated or too low temperatures can lead to tissue damage, organ function failure and variations in the metabolism rhythms. As being temperature such a vital parameter in life, the regulation of body temperature or thermoregulation becomes a critical body function. Thermoregulation is a complex process that involves several thermal sensors located on the skin, tissues and different areas of the brain. The information collected by these bio-sensing units is processed by the hypothalamus so that different processes of heat generation, conservation, dissipation or redistribution are triggered accordingly to the internal and external temperature. With all of this, the normal thermoregulation process sets the body core temperature in the range of 36.4 °C to 37.3 °C [81]. Detecting changes outside this normal window through continuous monitoring of the patient's core temperature is an essential tool for physicians since it can be used for early response whenever a set threshold has been reached.

Apart from the uses in health sciences, continuous temperature monitoring is also crucial for the electronics of an IMS. First, as described in Section 7.2.3, a significant problem associated with piezoresistive sensors (as well as other types of sensing elements) is their temperature sensitivity. Given these issues, for providing meaningful information from a piezoresistive transducer, the temperature should also be taken with high accuracy so that correction can be applied to the measurements. Furthermore, electronics in an IMS can produce heat during operation, which not only reduces their performance but also could result in a risk to the tissue surrounding the device [82] if the generated heat is high. Consequently, the monitoring of the temperature in the core elements of an IMS is a tool to keep the electronics within safe limits.

4.1 Temperature transducers

Temperature sensing history goes back centuries when scientists realised that specific material properties changes due to heat could be used to estimate the ambient or the temperature of a subject. It is recorded that the first device used to measure ambient temperature was invented by Galileo Galilei (XVI century) [83]. After this invention, several developments on temperature sensing devices lead to Daniel Gabriel Fahrenheit and Anders Celsius to develop their respective scales. A common factor is that all these developments were done with devices based on thermal expansion of liquids or metal pieces bonded together.

The demonstration of the thermoelectric effect by Thomas Johann Seebeck in 1820 [84] opened the doors for the estimation of temperature through electric and electronic devices. Since then, the study of the relationship between electrical material properties and temperature has lead to the development of more sophisticated temperature transducers. Analogue temperature sensors can be categorised into resistive and thermoelectric thermometers.

The most basic electric parameter used to measure temperature is the electrical resistance of conductors and semiconductors. Certain materials provide highly accurate and reproducible relationships between the temperature and its resistance. Thermistors and Resistance Temperature Detectors (RTD) belong to this category. RTD are fabricated with metals, making them useful for the measurement of large temperature ranges. In the other hand, Thermistors, made of ceramics or polymers, have a more limited temperature range but with a higher resolution than RTD [85].

As mentioned, a second type of analogue temperature transducers are those based on the Seebeck or thermoelectric effect. This effect describes that there is a current flow in a closed loop made of two wires of different conductive materials, anytime there is a difference of temperature between the two junctions (connecting the wires). In the case of having only one junction between the wires (i.e., the loop is not closed), a voltage is generated at the junction in the presence of a temperature gradient along the wires. This type of device is called a thermocouple [83].

The typical analogue thermal sensors such as thermocouples set the foundations to the electrical measurement of temperature. However, these devices pose restrictions to integration in miniature IMS. With the advent of microelectronics, researchers have used the properties of semiconductors to realise different types of transducers, being temperature sensing elements one of them. The combination of the transducer with its driving and data processing circuitry on a single chip has made integrated temperature sensors widely used in the last decades.

4.2 Integrated temperature transducer design

On-chip temperature sensing is a desired feature when developing IMS. The use of integrated temperature transducers allows area reduction since it does not require an extra component and the associated routing and bonding to the implant circuit board. Furthermore, several sensors can be placed on-chip so that they can serve multiple purposes. A requisite, however, is to design a temperature measurement system that provides high accuracy reading while keeping a low power consumption and low area utilisation.

4.2.1 On-chip sensing methods

When designing integrated temperature units, several options are available on standard CMOS technologies. Each type of element found on a CMOS technology has a different dependency on the temperature. Some of the integrated devices that can be used for sensing temperature are:

- **Resistors:** The magnitude and the sign of their temperature coefficient depends on the way the resistor is realised [86]. Figure 4.1 shows the implementation of resistors in a standard CMOS process. The following is a summary of the main characteristics of integrated CMOS resistors:

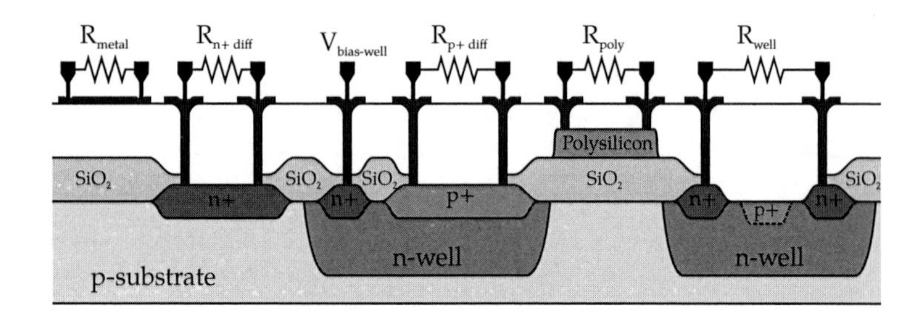

FIGURE 4.1: Simplified view of the implementation of resistors in a standard CMOS process.

- **Metal resistors**, made from a strip of interconnect metal (R_{metal} in Figure 4.1), typically present large temperature coefficients [87]. However, their main disadvantage is that their sheet-resistance is low, and then only small resistance values can be achieved in a reasonable area, which translates into high power consumption.
- **Diffusion resistors**, formed by shallow n+ or p+ implants ($R_{\text{n+diff}}$ and $R_{\text{p+diff}}$ in Figure 4.1). The temperature coefficient on these devices is comparable to that of metal resistors. However, the bias voltages affect the resistance by modulating their thickness [87].
- **Polysilicon resistors** (R_{poly} in Figure 4.1) temperature coefficient sign can be chosen by exposing the material to the appropriate implant [86]. The sheet resistance is considerable, but they suffer from large pink noise effects [87]. Also, their resistance value has a small dependency on the biasing voltage.
- **Well resistors** (R_{well} in Figure 4.1), which are formed by a low doping n-well, typically offer the highest sheet resistance [87] with a large positive temperature dependency. Furthermore, adding a p+ implant layer on top of the resistor increases its resistance (called *pinch resistor* [86]). However, the biasing voltage dependency of these resistors is large.

- **CMOS transistors:** The threshold voltage [88], subthreshold leakage current [89] and the source to drain on-resistance (mobility variations) [59] are parameters from CMOS devices that are dependent on the temperature. A typical task for microelectronics designers is to cancel the variations on these parameters through careful design and matching;

however, under the right conditions, they can be exploited to measure temperature. Two of these effects are:

- **Threshold voltage:** The threshold voltage in MOS devices presents a nearly linear sensitivity to temperature. This relationship is proportional to the temperature change and, for instance, in the BSIM-4 model is given by [88]:

$$V_{\text{th}}(T) = V_{\text{th}}(T_{\text{NOM}}) + \left(K_{\text{T1}} + \frac{K_{\text{T1L}}}{L_{\text{eff}}} + K_{\text{T2}} V_{\text{bs,eff}}\right)\left(\frac{T}{T_{\text{NOM}}} - 1\right), \tag{4.1}$$

  where T and T_{NOM} are the absolute and nominal absolute (the temperature at which the model parameters are extracted) temperature in Kelvin, respectively. Also, L_{eff} is the effective-length, $V_{\text{bs,eff}}$ is the effective bulk-source voltage, and parameters K_{T1}, K_{T1L} and K_{T2} are constants.

- **Subthreshold leakage current:** This technique is capturing interest in newer CMOS technologies since the leakage current has increased with the reduction of the minimum features. From the different components that contribute to the leakage current, the subthreshold conduction dominates. In this way, the subthreshold leakage current is modelled as [90]:

$$I_{\text{d,st}}(T) = \mu_0 C_{\text{ox}} \frac{W}{L} \left(\frac{kT}{q}\right)^2 e^{1.8} e^{\frac{V_{\text{gs}} - V_{\text{th}}(T)}{nkT/q}} \left(1 - e^{-\frac{V_{\text{ds}}}{kT/q}}\right), \tag{4.2}$$

  where n is the subthreshold slope, μ_0 is the zero bias carrier mobility, and $V_{\text{th}}(T)$ is the threshold voltage (which also varies with temperature). This expression can be approximated to an exponential model, where the leakage varies in a positive exponential way with the temperature [90].

- **Parasitic Bipolar Junction Transistors (BJT):** These parasitic devices are formed by two consecutive PN junctions in a CMOS device. In a typical application, these devices are avoided by adequately biasing the substrate and the different p-wells across the design (or even n-wells on multi-well processes). However, for some applications such as bandgap voltage references or temperature sensing, these parasitic bipolar transistors can be used. Figure 4.2 shows some examples of BJTs realisations

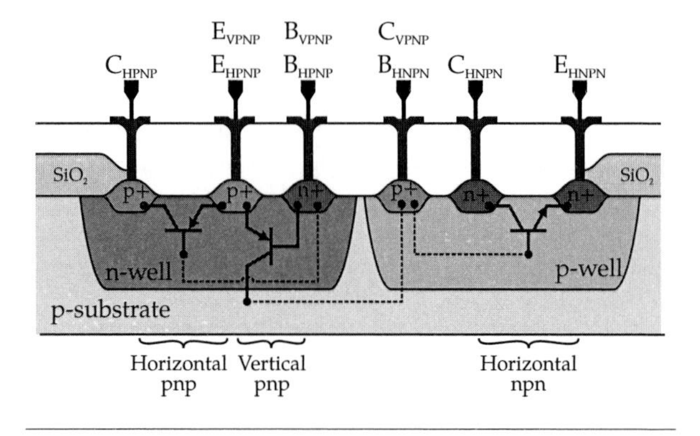

FIGURE 4.2: Simplified diagram depicting the parasitic bipolar transistors in a standard CMOS process.

in a standard CMOS process. Both PNP and NPN BJTs can be implemented using standard CMOS technology. Compared to the use of CMOS transistors, these devices offer better temperature characteristics, low stress-effects, and their physics are reliable and predictable (which is essential for industrial applications) [91, 92]. On bipolar transistors, two characteristic voltages play a role in the temperature measurement, the silicon bandgap voltage and the thermal voltage [86].

4.2.2 Implementation of temperature sensing unit

In this work, a temperature sensing unit was developed using vertical PNP BJT. Lateral BJT were not used since their characteristics get degraded due to parasitic vertical BJT [93]. BJT were chosen, given their reliability and low effects due to stress [91].

Figure 4.3.a shows a PNP-BJT diode-connected biased by a current reference circuit. Under this configuration, the emitter-base voltage V_{EB} presents a Complementary to absolute temperature behaviour [92] described by [94]:

$$V_{\mathrm{EB}} = V_{\mathrm{G0}}\left(1 - \frac{T}{T_0}\right) + V_{\mathrm{EB0}}\left(\frac{T}{T_0}\right) + \frac{\gamma_{\mathrm{tc}} k_{\mathrm{B}} T}{q}\ln\left(\frac{T}{T_0}\right) + \frac{k_{\mathrm{B}} T}{q}\ln\left(\frac{J_{\mathrm{C}}}{J_{\mathrm{C0}}}\right), \tag{4.3}$$

where T is the temperature in Kelvin, V_{G0} is the bandgap voltage of silicon at 0 K (equal to 1.206 V), γ_{tc} is a process-dependent temperature-constant, and J_{C} is the collector current density at temperature T. Additionally, V_{EB0} and J_{C0} are the V_{EB} and the collector current density at a reference temperature

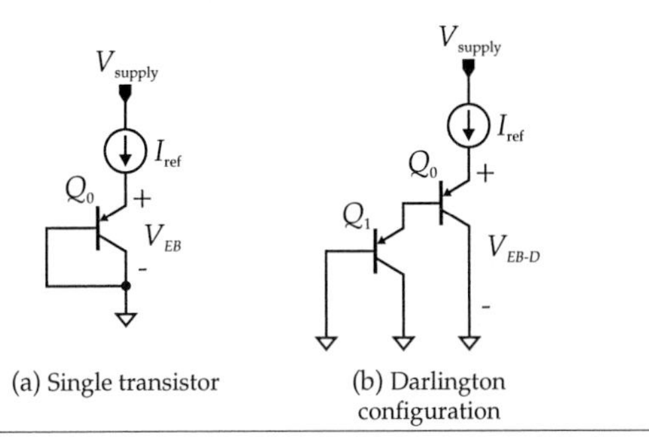

(a) Single transistor

(b) Darlington configuration

FIGURE 4.3: Temperature sensing element based on Diode connected PNP-BJT.

T_0, respectively. The expression for V_{EB} shows non-linearity with respect to the temperature, as well as a dependency on the biasing conditions and the transistor sizing.

On Equation 4.3, the last term is dominant. Hence, an approximation for the temperature coefficient for a single diode-connected BJT biased with a constant emitter current I_{ref} is given by [95]:

$$\frac{\partial V_{\mathrm{EB}}}{\partial T} = \frac{V_{\mathrm{EB}} - (4+m)k_{\mathrm{B}}Tq^{-1} - E_{\mathrm{g}}q^{-1}}{T}, \tag{4.4}$$

where E_{g} is the silicon band-gap energy ($\approx 1.11\,\mathrm{eV}$) and $m \approx 3/2$. Figure 4.4 shows the temperature dependency, for different biasing currents, of the emitter-base voltage of the diode-connected PNP-BJT transistor from Figure 4.3.a. These curves are based on a simulation with a vertical PNP-BJT in 180 nm CMOS technology. Here is possible to see the effect on the slopes due to biasing (including the error due to process mismatch).

The temperature sensitivity of the configuration in Figure 4.3.a is promising, however by including and extra BJT and using a simple Darlington configuration, as in Figure 4.3.b, the sensitivity can be improved. In the case of this device, the equivalent emitter to base voltage is roughly twice the V_{EB} of a single BJT. Therefore, the temperature coefficient can be approximated to:

$$\frac{\partial V_{\mathrm{EB,d}}}{\partial T} = 2\left(\frac{V_{\mathrm{EB,d}} - (4+m)k_{\mathrm{B}}Tq^{-1} - E_{\mathrm{g}}q^{-1}}{T}\right), \tag{4.5}$$

which represents approximately a doubling of the temperature sensitivity of the device. Figure 4.5.a shows a temperature sweep for the Darlington element

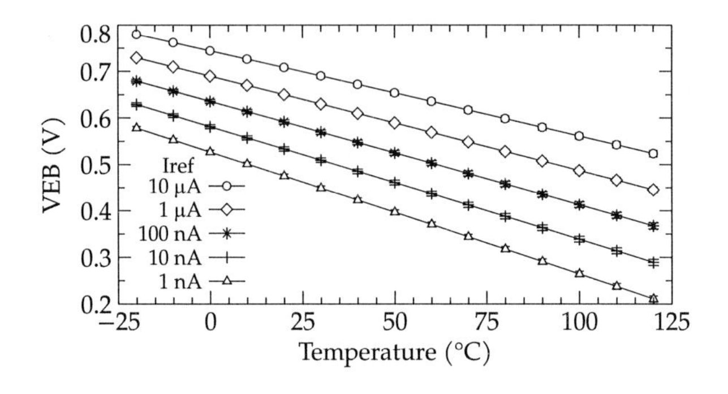

FIGURE 4.4: Emitter-base voltage V_{EB} vs Temperature for various biasing currents for a diode-connected PNP-BJT in CMOS 180 nm technology.

from Figure 4.3.b. Under this configuration, the temperature sensitivity is high as can be appreciated in Figure 4.5.b; however, for large temperature ranges, the variation in sensitivity is an issue. Nevertheless, for the use in an IMS, this should not be a problem since the temperature range is limited to a few degrees around the typical body temperature. Furthermore, as Figure 4.5.a shows, the output voltage of the sensing unit has a higher magnitude when compared with the single BJT circuit, which in turn translates in a higher limit to the minimum supply voltage for the IMS.

A consequence of Equation 4.5 is that for this temperature sensing method, it is crucial to provide a stable collector current to the darling pair. Therefore, any implementation requires a PVT-independent current reference to provide a stable I_{ref} (Figure 4.3.b).

4.3 Implementation and results

Figure 4.6 shows the schematic view of the implemented temperature sensing unit. The system consists of a current reference, a current mirror and the Darlington pair (from Figure 4.3.b). Regarding the current reference circuit, it is based on the design presented in Appendix A. In this design, the transistor M_{N0} and M_{N1} operate in saturation and linear regions, respectively. Additionally, M_{N3}, M_{P4}, and M_{P5} are used as switches for the startup circuitry. The rest of MOS transistors operate in the subthreshold region. Following a similar approach as in Appendix A, it is possible to size the transistors to achieve a PVT current reference.

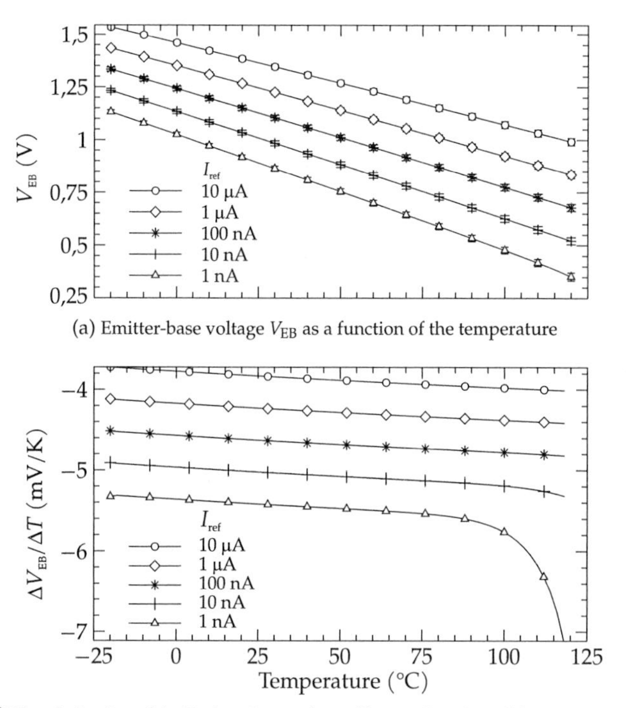

(a) Emitter-base voltage V_{EB} as a function of the temperature

(b) First derivative of the Emitter-base voltage V_{EB} as a function of the temperature.

FIGURE 4.5: Temperature dependency for a diode-connected PNP-Darlington configuration in CMOS 180 nm technology under different biasing currents.

It was decided to bias the Darlington pair with a current close to 100 nA. As shown in Figure 4.5, for currents around 100 nA the variation temperature coefficient of this sensing element is minimal, offering also a linear behaviour for a broader temperature range than the resulting from lower biasing currents. Furthermore, for this biasing condition, the sensitivity magnitude is still higher than 4 mV °C^{-1}.

The designed temperature sensing module was implemented in 180 nm CMOS technology. About the implemented current reference circuit, simulations resulted in an average current of 124.88 nA (at 37 °C) with a standard deviation of 227 pA. Furthermore, in the temperature range of interest (i.e., an IMS) from 32 °C to 42 °C, the output current has a temperature coefficient of −22.33 pA °C^{-1}.

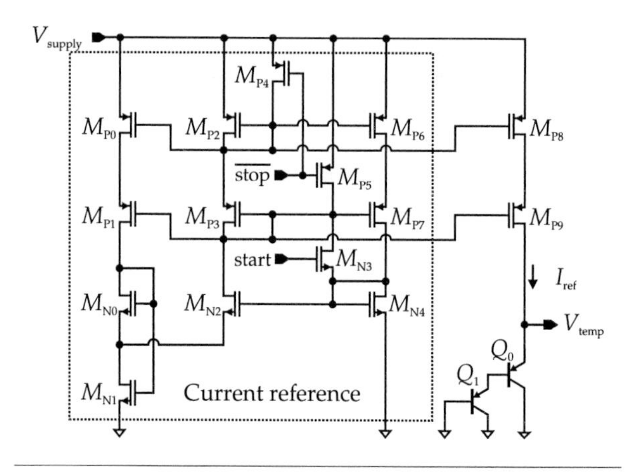

FIGURE 4.6: Schematic view of the implemented temperature sensing unit.

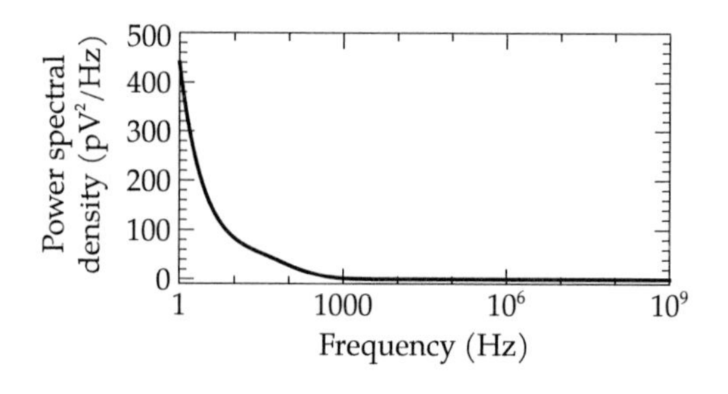

FIGURE 4.7: Simulated noise power spectral density at the temperature sensor output.

The full temperature sensing module simulation exhibited an average slope $-4.890\,\mathrm{mV\,°C^{-1}}$ in the range 32 °C to 42 °C. This sensitivity value has a standard deviation of 29.311 µV due to process and mismatch variations. Moreover, Figure 4.7 shows the power spectral density for this sensor unit. From this curve, the total uncertainty obtained for a bandwidth of 1 kHz is $1.182 \times 10^{-8}\,\mathrm{V}^2$, which translates into a minimum detectable change in temperature of 0.022 °C. Finally, the simulations showed an average power consumption during operation of 1.123 µW for a supply of 1.8 V and at 37 °C.

The described system was fabricated as part of the test ASIC shown in Appendix B.2. Figure 4.8 shows an annotated micrograph of the implementation. The total area occupied by the temperature sensor unit is $0.012\,\mathrm{mm}^2$.

Five ASICs were packaged and tested. The test results are shown in Figure 4.9. From the experiments, it was determined an average temperature sensitivity of $-4.7463\,\mathrm{mV\,°C^{-1}}$ (117.56 ppm) with a standard deviation of $55.8\,\mathrm{\mu V\,°C^{-1}}$. Furthermore, the maximum offset difference between the ICs outputs is 18.59 mV. Finally, the average power consumption, during operation, was measured at 927 nW.

The temperature sensitivity achieved and the low power and area consumption of the presented transducer, makes it a good candidate for the temperature reading in IMS.

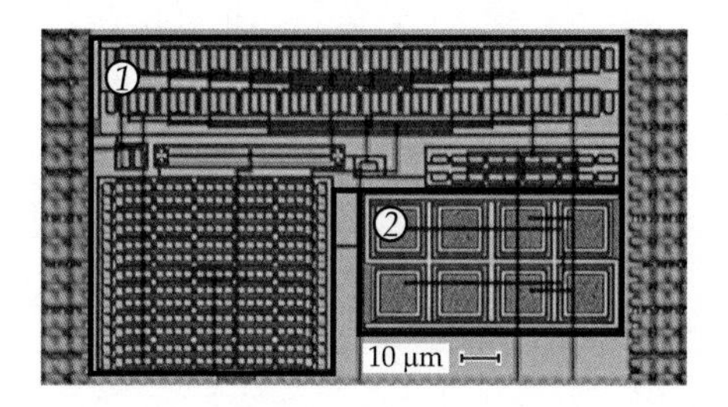

FIGURE 4.8: Annotated micrograph of the temperature transducer implemented in 180 nm CMOS technology. 1. Current reference, 2.BJT Darlington Pair.

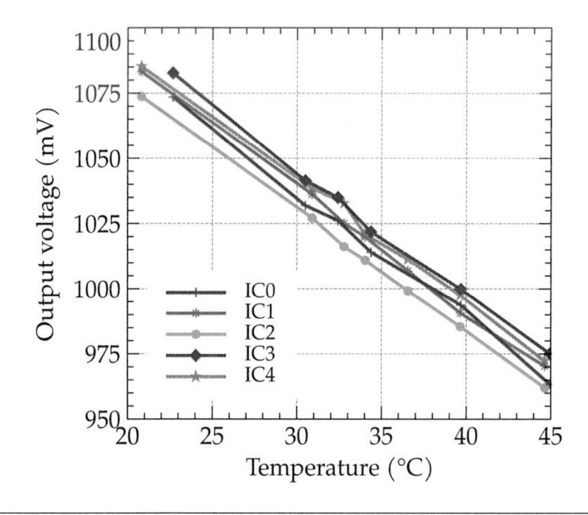

FIGURE 4.9: Experimental results for the temperature transducer implemented in 180 nm CMOS technology.

Chapter 5

Timing

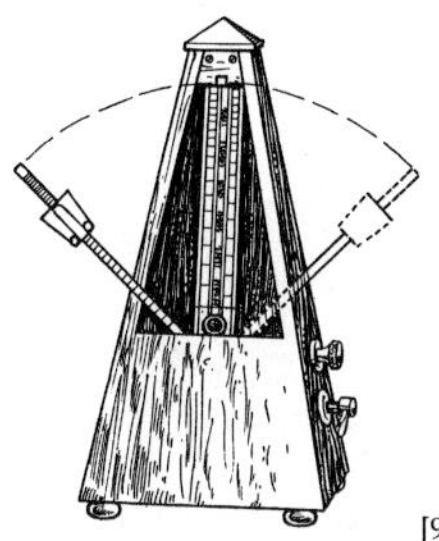

[96]

Timing and clock generation units are required by a broad set of electronic devices in several fields, including medical applications. On the case of timing, these units should be designed with low deviation in order to provide accurate timestamps for the process under observation. For clock units, the variation tolerance depends on the application; if the clock unit is used on a data converter, high accuracy is required (as in Section 3.2.2.2). In contrast, if the unit handles a low-frequency control unit, some deviation can be handled anytime the performance of the device is not compromised.

For the low-power low-data rate pressure monitoring medical devices described in this work, the timing has a high impact on the device power budget and usability. The timing unit is part of the power management unit in Figure 2.1. The timing is one of the few blocks that is permanently powered, and hence its power consumption has to be optimised for maximising the system autonomy. However, inaccuracy on the time counting of this unit can lead to data interpretation problems once the information has been recovered from the implant. In the case of the main-clock unit (used to drive the control unit), the accuracy is in frequency is not critical since it is powered only during the sampling process, and it does not affect any of the data converters or sampling time.

5.1 Low power timer design [97]

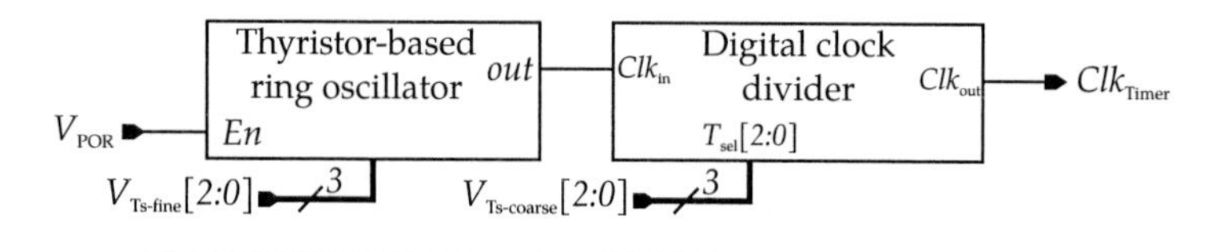

FIGURE 5.1: Block diagram of the timer unit.

This work proposes a re-configurable low power timer based on a thyristor ring oscillator, as shown in Figure 5.1. The vantage of this architecture is that few thyristor elements are required in order to produce long delays which translates into small area utilisation and reductions on power consumption. Also, the option to configure the final timer period, allows for this unit to be used in multiple applications.

5.1.1 Re-configurable delay thyristor-based unit cell

Low-frequency timing requires the use of efficient delay elements for producing long periods. Also, the circuits have to be designed in such a way that static power is minimised. In section Section 3.2.2.2, the thyristor element was introduced as a construction block that can produce large delays with a reduced design complexity. As shown in Figure 5.2, the thyristor element can be adapted to depend only on leakage currents and therefore, the current reference circuit is not required. This unit cell is based on the thyristor in Figure 3.20, and in contrast to the design in Section 3.2.2.2, the leakage current value is crucial in this circuit.

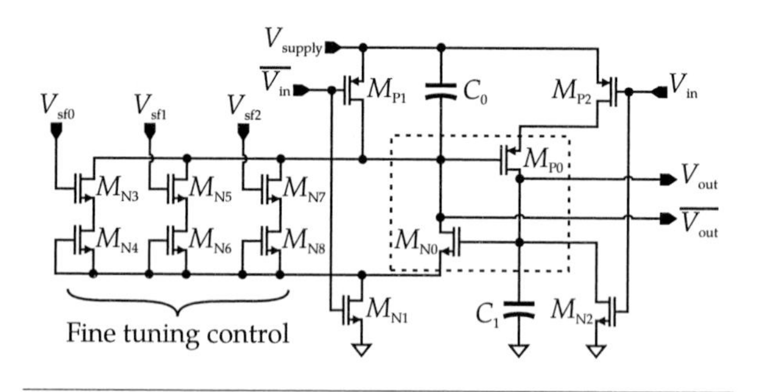

FIGURE 5.2: Schematic view of the thyristor-based delay cell with fine tuning-control.

As shown in Figure 5.2, the thyristor unit is formed by transistors M_{N0} and M_{P0} connected in a positive feedback loop (enclosed in the dotted line box in Figure 5.2). Transistors M_{P1} and M_{N2} are used to force the thyristor element to its *off* state when V_{in} and $\overline{V_{in}}$ are equal to V_{supply} and ground, respectively. This first phase is depicted in the diagram in Figure 5.3. The second phase is triggered by pulling V_{in} to ground (and therefore $\overline{V_{in}}$ to V_{supply}). This trigger signal causes transistors M_{N1} and M_{P2} to close (while M_{P1} and M_{N2} are opened), which creates a path that slowly charges C_1 towards V_{supply} through the leakage current of M_{P0}, as well the discharges the node $\overline{V_{out}}$ to ground (the voltage difference between the plates of C_0 is V_{supply}). After this, the thyristor enters its *on* state. The time Δt_{dc} (shown in Figure 5.3) taken by this unit cell to transition between states after V_{in} is pulled to low is given by:

$$\Delta t_{dc} = \frac{C_{eq-out}}{I_{leak-MP0} - I_{leak-MN2}} V_{thn} , \tag{5.1}$$

where C_{eq-out} is the equivalent capacitance seen in node V_{out} and $I_{leak-MX}$ is the leakage current of transistor M_X. During these transition phase, the transistors are biased in the subthreshold region [98], which means that the drain current (leakage) is computed as [99]:

$$I_D = 2n\mu C'_{ox} \frac{W}{L} V_T^2 e^{\frac{V_G - V_{th}}{nV_T}} \left(e^{\frac{-V_S}{V_T}} - e^{\frac{-V_D}{V_T}} \right) , \tag{5.2}$$

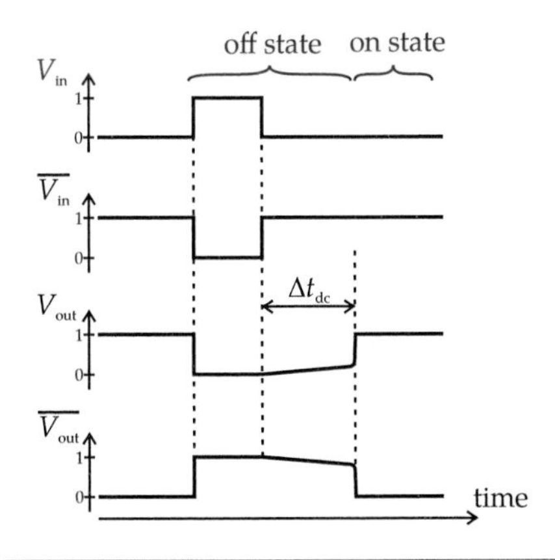

FIGURE 5.3: Main signal waveforms for the leakage-based thyristor unit cell.

which shows the dependency of the leakage current on the width (W) and length (L) of the transistors channel. Then Equations 5.1 and 5.2 can be used to define the sizing of the transistors in the delay cell, as well the capacitance value for C_0 and C_1, based on the timing requirements.

A feature added to the cell in Figure 5.2 is the option to tune the time delay Δt_{dc}. This fine-tuning is done using set of transistors in *off* state ($V_{\mathrm{GS}} = 0\ V$) that can be connected (or disconnected) in parallel to transistor M_{N0} (part of the thyristor core). The channel length for transistors M_{N4}, M_{N6} and M_{N8} is the same as of M_{N0}; however, their width is a binary-weighted multiple of M_{N0} channel width. In this way, $W_{\mathrm{MN4}} = W_{\mathrm{MN0}}$, $W_{\mathrm{MN6}} = 2 \times W_{\mathrm{MN0}}$ and $W_{\mathrm{MN8}} = 4 \times W_{\mathrm{MN0}}$. The connection of these transistors is handled by the control bus $V_{\mathrm{sf}}[2,0]$.

5.1.2 Thyristor-based ring oscillator

A set of delay cell (as those presented in Figure 5.2) can be combined to form a ring oscillator, as shown in Figure 5.4. The delay provided on each of the $N_{\mathrm{dc-timer}}$ stages is added to produce the ring oscillator period $T_{\mathrm{osc-timer}}$ as:

$$T_{\mathrm{osc-timer}} = N_{\mathrm{dc-timer}}\, t_{\mathrm{dc}} + \delta_{\mathrm{digital}}\,, \tag{5.3}$$

where $\delta_{\mathrm{digital}}$ is the delay on the timer enable logic (digital blocks in Figure 5.4). The enable signal has to be provided by a Power-on-Reset (PoR) block present in the implantable system. With this enable logic, the timer output is placed on a known state (V_{out} high and $\overline{V_{\mathrm{out}}}$ low) before operation.

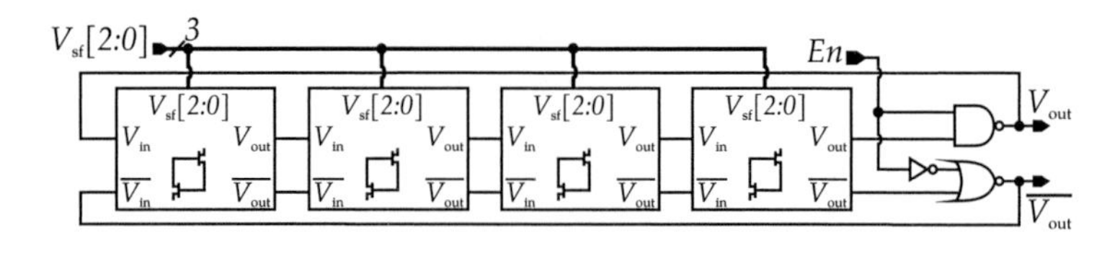

FIGURE 5.4: Thyristor-based ring oscillator block diagram.

5.1.3 Digital clock divider

As shown in Figure 5.1, a configurable clock divider block is included in the timer design. This unit provides further flexibility to the clock unit to adjust in large steps the frequency of the timer. A digital bus $V_{\mathrm{Ts-coarse}}[2:0]$ is used to select among a set of frequency division presets. The digital code of each preset does not necessarily correspond to the binary word on the control bus. However, it can be chosen based on the requirements of different scenarios where the implantable device is going to be used.

5.2 Control system clock generation and gating [97]

The timer unit presented in Section 5.1 is used for generating long delays for sleep cycle management. However, the frequency of this signal is too low for driving the control unit of the implant. Due to this, a secondary oscillator unit is required for running the digital blocks that form the main control module. In this work, a clock management unit is proposed, as shown in Figure 5.5. In this unit, the clock signal is generated by a current controlled oscillator (CCO) based on the use of thyristor elements. The frequency of this oscillator is set to a fixed value by a low power current reference designed as in Appendix A. Furthermore, the clock gating unit present in the diagram in Figure 5.5 is used to enable the clock by using the signal from the timer (Section 5.1) and also to receive a disable signal generated by the control unit once this one has finished all its tasks.

5.2.1 Thyristor-based current controlled oscillator

In Section 3.2.2.2, the thyristor element was presented as a low power device able to provide a controllable time transition delay between its two stable states. As with the CTC unit cell, the thyristor concept can be adapted to produce a delay that depends on the capacitance in the thyristor nodes (P_{trig} and N_{trig} in Figure 3.21.a) and the discharging current. With this in mind, and based on the work in [67], the delay cell shown in Figure 5.6.a can be used as a building block for low-frequency clock generation.

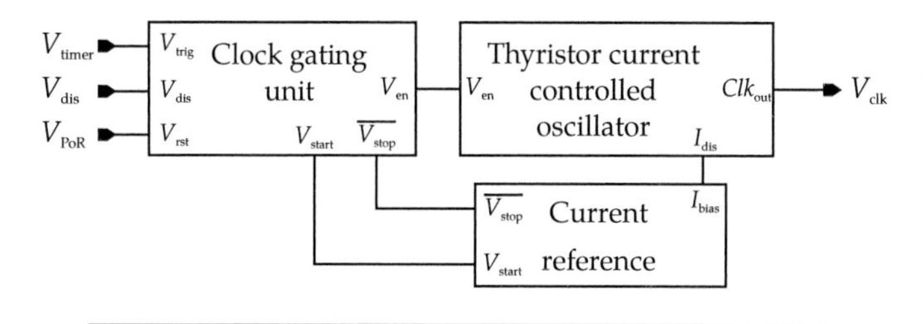

FIGURE 5.5: Block diagram of the Clock management unit.

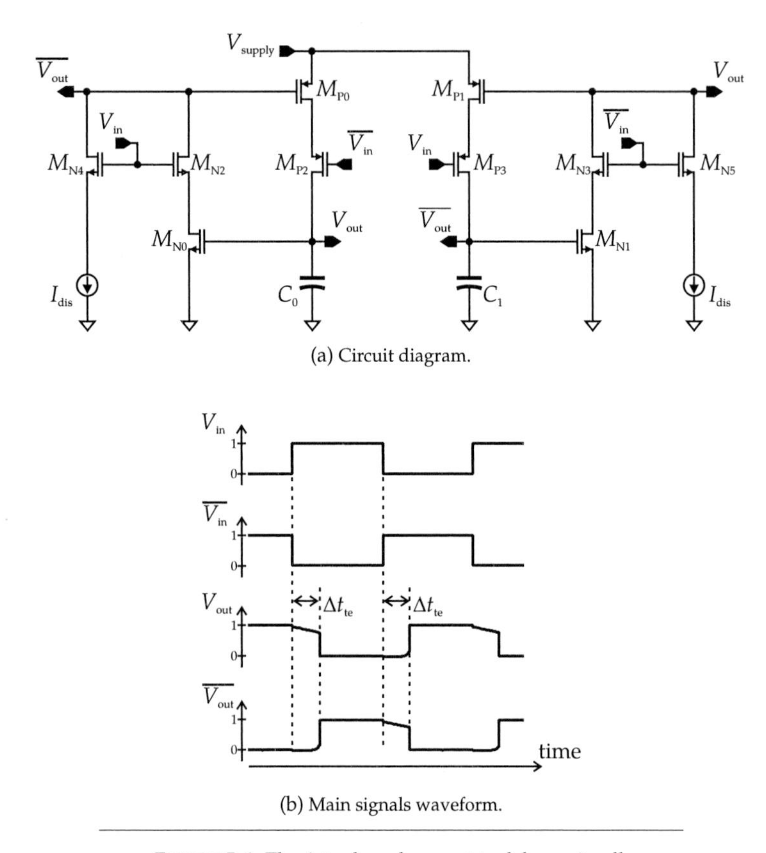

(a) Circuit diagram.

(b) Main signals waveform.

FIGURE 5.6: Thyristor-based current to delay unit cell.

As shown in Figure 5.6.b, the unit cell produces delays at both edges of the signal V_{in} (and the complementary signal $\overline{V_{\text{in}}}$). By defining the capacitors in $C_0 = C$ and $C_1 = C$ as the equivalent node capacitance at the nodes V_{out} and $\overline{V_{\text{out}}}$, respectively, and using Equation 3.35 the delay seen after an edge can be calculated as:

$$t_{\text{te}} = \frac{CV_{\text{thp}}}{I_{\text{dis}}} + \sqrt[3]{\frac{6C^3}{\kappa_{\text{p}} I_{\text{dis}}^2} V_{\text{thn}}} + \delta t\,. \tag{5.4}$$

the matching between the elements on each branch and the value of the equivalent capacitance on the output nodes are crucial to keep valid the previous expression.

Using these unit cells, it possible to implement an N-stage ring oscillator in the same way as in Figure 5.4; however, in this case, the oscillator period has to be computed as:

$$T_{\mathrm{clk}} = 2\,N\,t_{\mathrm{te}} + \delta_{\mathrm{digital}}\,. \tag{5.5}$$

Equations 5.4 and 5.5 can be used as design criteria for this type of oscillator.

5.2.2 Clock gating unit

The proposed clock gating unit is presented in Figure 5.7.a. This block links the timer described in Section 5.1 and the clock generator from section Section 5.2. As shown in Figure 5.5, the block receives as input the timer output signal V_{timer} (as well the reset signal from the system PoR unit) and generates the required signals for the clock and current reference units.

The waveforms in Figure 5.7.b show the relationship between the main signals in the clock gating unit. At startup, the PoR block in the IMS-ASIC system is low, which is used by this unit to set all the internal registers to a stable reset state. Once the signal V_{PoR} is latched to high, the system is ready to operate. The clock gating block outputs (V_{start}, V_{stop} and V_{en}) remain low until the next positive edge of the timer signal V_{timer}.

The positive edge of V_{timer} triggers the clock initialisation sequence. The signal V_{stop} is first generated by the flip-flop 3 in Figure 5.7.a. After a short delay, the signal V_{start} is generated, the pulse width of this signal is set by the delay element 4 (Figure 5.7.a). These two signals are used in the startup circuitry of the current reference that sets the discharging currents of the thyristor-CCO. As described in Appendix A, it takes some time for the current reference to stabilise after the V_{start} pulse, because of this, the delay element 6 in Figure 5.7.a is in the path of V_{en} signal. In this way, a stable clock signal V_{clk} for the main digital control is generated. A clock disable signal V_{dis} is provided in order to turn-off the clock generation once the main digital control unit finished its tasks and V_{clk} is not required anymore. After a short delay from the positive edge of V_{dis}, all signals return to low, causing the clock to stop and the current reference to be turned off.

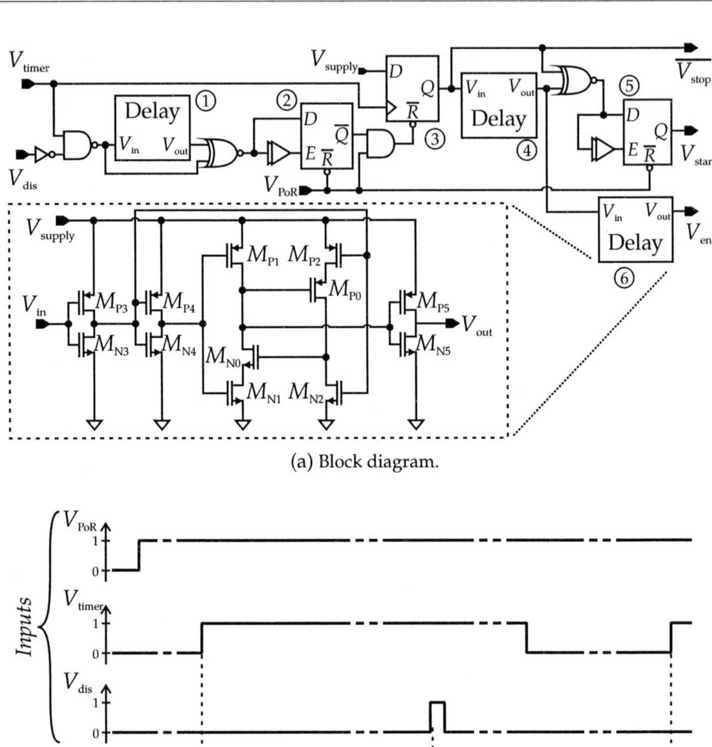

(a) Block diagram.

(b) Main signals waveform.

FIGURE 5.7: Clock gating unit.

5.3 Timing unit implementation and results [97]

In order to prove the concept, the timing unit described in this chapter was implemented as part of a test chip (Appendix B.1). The fabricated unit micrograph is shown in Figure 5.8. In the case of the thyristor-based timer, the area utilised was 0.025 mm^2, while the clock generation unit occupies 0.0344 mm^2. For test purposes, ten sample ASICs were packaged (in a ceramic JLCC package) and placed in a PCB that allowed access to the main pins of the system. A stable regulated power supply was used to ensure low noise measurements. For current consumption readings, a commercial sub-femtoampere meter was used.

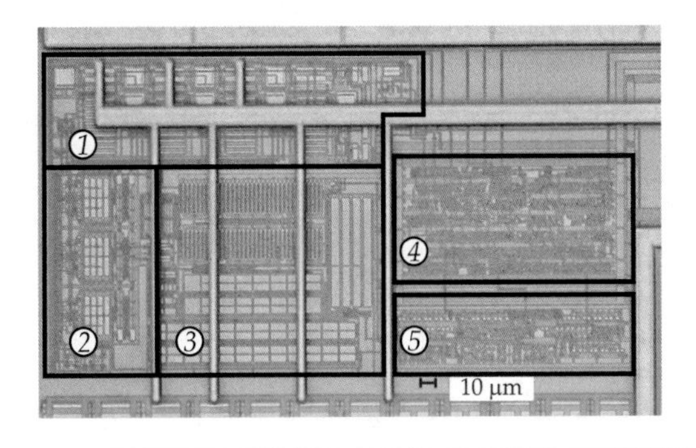

FIGURE 5.8: Annotated micrograph of the timing unit implemented in 350 nm CMOS technology. 1. Thyristor-based timer, 2. Thyristor-based current-controlled oscillator, 3. Current reference, 4. Clock divider, 5. Clock gating logic.

5.3.1 Timer unit results

For the timer tests, a setup comprising the test ICs, a stable power supply and controlled temperature chamber was set. For measuring the period, a digital oscilloscope working as data logger with a USB interface to a PC was used. Figure 5.9 presents the results from long-term test performed using the test IC; these tests were done at a temperature of 37 °C and a supply of 3.3 V. The resulting average period is then 32.45 s with a standard deviation of 0.63 s. Furthermore, under these conditions, the timer unit drains, on average, 600 pA of current (with a standard deviation of 54.21 pA).

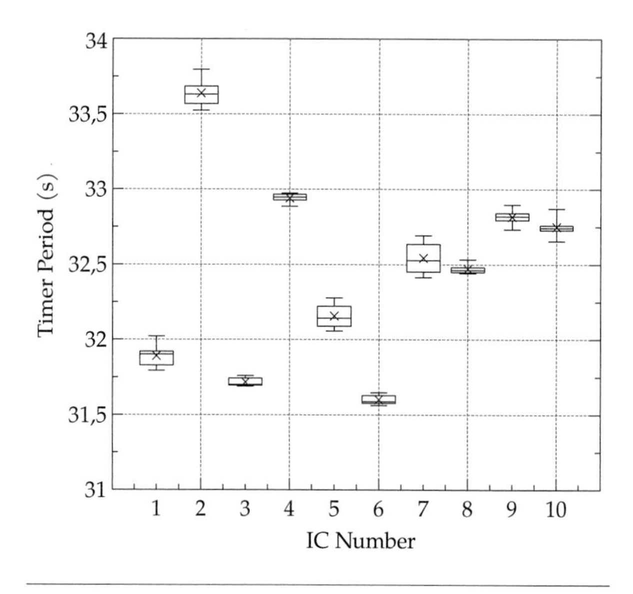

FIGURE 5.9: Timer period measured for the ten sample ICs at 37 °C, 3.3 V supply voltage and minimum clock division setting.

The temperature dependency of the timer period was verified by measuring several cycles for different temperatures in the range 36 °C to 41 °C. The tests result shows that the impact over the timer period due to temperature has a magnitude of $-0.685\,\mathrm{s\,°C^{-1}}$. Additionally, it was found that for this unit, the period is also dependent on the supply voltage with a variation of 324.2 ms per 100 mV of change. This last parameter is required to define the specifications of the power supply for the timer so that the period variations are limited.

The process variations that cause the different periods seen in Figure 5.9 can be corrected by using the trimming mechanism shown in Figure 5.2. Simulations showed that for this implementation, the period could be changed in steps of 1.42 s per each step of the trimming logic.

The low power consumption, reduced area, and low drift, together with the option of trimming any offset, makes this unit a good option for the timekeeping on IMSs with low power budgets and low data rate requirements.

5.3.2 Clock unit results

As with the timer unit, the clock gating and generation unit was fabricated as part of a test ASIC (Appendix B.1). The generated clock period was measured in a long-term test (a similar approach as used for the timer). A peculiarity of this test is that the timer is active only for a short time after enabled (by the positive edge of the timer signal). For this reason, the measurement per chip corresponds to the average clock period for several of these cycles. Figure 5.10 shows the measured clock frequency on each of the tested ICs.

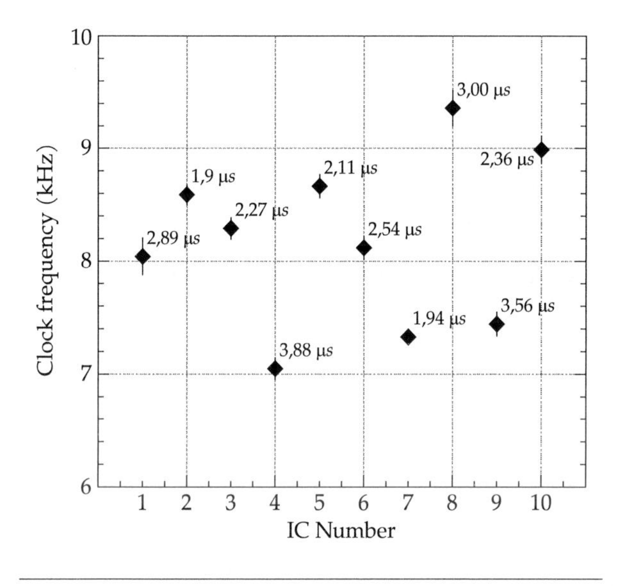

FIGURE 5.10: Clock frequency measured (and associated RMS Jitter) for the ten sample ICs at 37 °C and 3.3 V supply voltage.

From the measurements taken from the clock generation unit, it was found that the average frequency was 8.19 kHz with a standard deviation of 93.6 Hz. The average Jitter resulted in 2.64 µs (with a standard deviation of 0.68 µs), which is equivalent to 2.46 % of the average period. Furthermore, part of the metrics that define the stability of the oscillator is the sensitivity to temperature and supply variations. For the implemented design, it was determined an average temperature coefficient of 1018 ppm/°C and a sensitivity to changes in the power supply of 1.1 % V^{-1}.

In the case of the clock gating unit, an important parameter is the delay between the trigger signal and the clock generation. As described previously, this delay allows for proper initialisation and settling of the current used to bias the thyristor-based oscillator. A sample of the measurement of this delay is shown in Figure 5.11. For the implemented system, and after running several log-term tests on the ten sample IC, it was found that the average delay has a value of 23.65 ms.

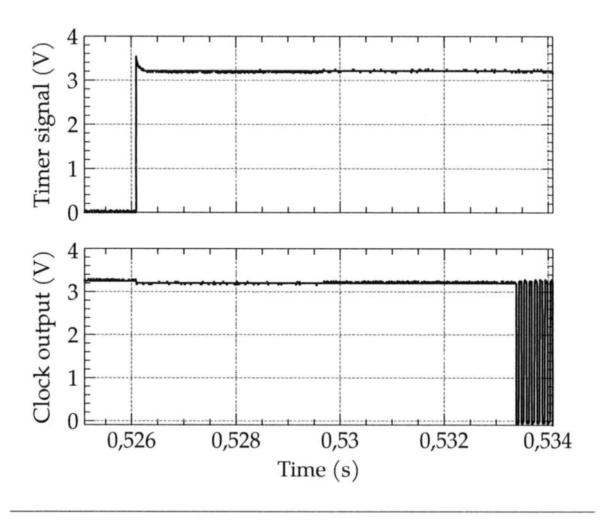

FIGURE 5.11: Sample measurement of the delay timer-positive-edge to clock-output.

Finally, the average measured power consumption for the clock generation and gating unit together was 1.29 nW. The resulting low power consumption and stable clock signal generated makes this unit suitable for providing the timing to a digital control unit on a miniaturised IMS.

The presented timing and clock generation unit displayed promising results in power and area utilisation. The reduced power consumed by these units (in the nanowatt range) makes them candidates for implantable systems with limited energy budgets. Furthermore, the reconfigurability of the timing unit period allows it to adapt to different application requirements.

Chapter 6

Device Encapsulation and Mechanics

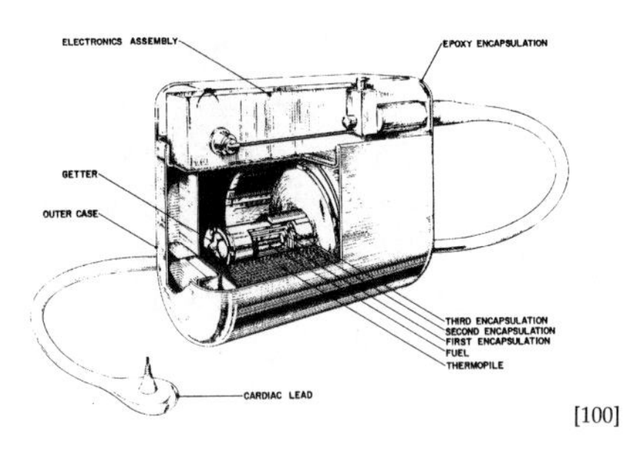

[100]

The previous chapters presented the electronics behind an IMS, yet developing and manufacturing such systems does not end there. The research and development of IMSs requires a multidisciplinary team. Physicians, health researches, and engineers from different fields such as electronics, computer, and materials sciences have to work together to successfully bring into reality a device that eventually will help in the research, prevention and healing of a disease. This chapter discusses three important matters related to the mechanics of the IMS, the device encapsulation, the manufacture of mechanical pieces and the generation of early prototypes or mockups.

6.1 Device encapsulation

The human body is a complex system in balance, and for its survival, it also represents a harsh environment for any invasive element. The electronic components in the IMS are in general bio-incompatible. Letting the wrong materials be in contact with the body internals can cause injuries to tissue or organs, exudation, acute and chronic inflammation of the surrounding areas

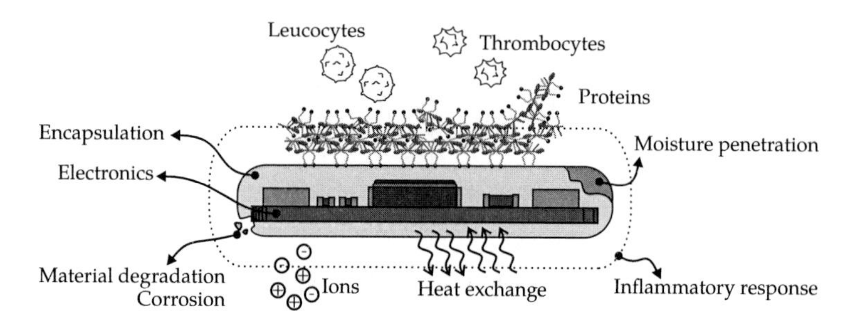

FIGURE 6.1: Some of the interactions and issues between the encapsulation of an IMS and the host body.

[7] among other reactions, that depending on the level of toxicity can cause permanent damages or even death. As well, once deployed, the implant is attacked by antigen and several biochemical reactions since this represents a foreign element [101]. These actions from the body can cause corrosion and damage to the more exposed parts of the implantable device. Furthermore, the fluids inside the body are loaded with ions, making them highly conductive; therefore if the IMS is not adequately isolated from these fluids, it can cause short circuits and malfunction.

A challenge for the research and development of IMS is to package the system to protect the device and the host body from harm. In this way, the material exposed to the tissue and fluids should not contain any toxic component, nor degrade into any compound that becomes incompatible with life or produces any undesired immune reaction [102]. Also, the package should support sterilisation [7], since this is a must before the device is implanted in the body [103]. A successful IMS encapsulation depends on the selection of the materials to be used, a mechanical design adapted to the implantation area, and a well-structured manufacturing procedure.

6.1.1 Materials for encapsulation

The expected use-time of a medical device allows to classify it into disposable and non-disposable. The products found in the disposable category are those that are used only once. These products are in contact with the patient for a limited amount of time and afterwards, are discarded. Some examples are syringes, catheters, bandages, among others [104]. In the other hand, non-disposable devices are used multiple times in one or several patients during its working life. Such devices are in contact with the body for prolonged periods, and this is the case of different diagnostic and treatment machines and instruments, prostheses, and implantable devices [104]. The material requirements for the non-disposable equipment are more challenging than those for disposable units.

In the non-disposable category, the selection of materials that can be used is limited to those with high mechanical, physical and chemical stability since long-term durability is primary. Material specifications such as bio-compatibility, resistance to sterilisation processes or chemicals, vary depending on the degree of contact with the body fluids, tissue and the exposition time to them. Regulations provide a framework to define the requirements for the materials used in an IMS so that they are safe for the patient or research subject [105]. Ultimately, the use of adequate materials for the encapsulation of the IMS will reduce the development of complications in the subject or the device, that might result in harm or death of the patient [106].

6.1.1.1 Requirements of encapsulation materials

As described previously, the specifications of encapsulation materials are a function of the application. The following is a list of requirements for materials used in IMS:

- **Bio-compatibility:** This is the most critical requirement for the encapsulation materials used in an IMS since they are in direct contact with body fluids and tissue. Following the IMS implantation, the body reaction depends on the interactions between the surface of the device and the surrounding biological elements. Biocompatibility can be defined as:

  > Biocompatibility refers to the ability of a biomaterial to perform its desired function with respect to a medical therapy, without eliciting any undesirable local or systemic effects in the recipient or beneficiary of that therapy, but generating the most appropriate beneficial cellular or tissue response in that specific situation, and optimising the clinically relevant performance of that therapy [107, p. 523]

  Thus for a material to be bio-compatible, it is indispensable to understand the healing response of the body at the location of implantation.

Furthermore, apart from the material composition and the device location, bio-compatibility depends on the fabrication, surface and macro-structure properties of the encapsulation [105].

- **Bio-stability:** This property is imperative for long-term implantable devices. A material is bio-stable if its chemical and structural properties do not show significant changes when immersed in a biological system for extensive periods [106]. Corrosion and wear, two symptoms of poor material bio-stability, have to be kept as low as possible. The evaluation of bio-stability needs to be done based on the characteristics at the expected IMS implantation location, as well as the therapies that the patient has to undergo (e.g. chemotherapy).In this way, the designer can acquire the knowledge on the electrolytes, biological, and chemical substances dissolved in the body fluids that will surround the device together with the local pH and temperature.
- **Thermal stability:** The encapsulation material has to withstand the constant body internal temperature. The average core temperature is considered 37 °C; however, it can vary largely depending on the health conditions and the therapies applied. For instance, when using hyperthermia for cancer treatment, the local temperature at application can go as high as 43.5 °C [18]. Moreover, care has to be taken when the materials have to be exposed to high temperatures during processing of the device or sterilisation procedures [104].
- **Mechanical stability:** The body is in continuous motion, and these produces mechanical stress to the implantable system. These forces, such as pressure and tension, cause wearing of the packaging. Therefore, the material selected has to offer enough mechanical strength so that the packaging hermiticity is not compromised and keeps protecting the device and the patient.
- **Electrical properties:** Some implantable devices would require that the encapsulating material provides electrical insulation from the body. However, on devices, such stimulators, part of the encapsulation has to allow for transfer of charge to the surrounding tissue. In this case, the designer has to care about the conductivity or dielectric constant of the material. [104]
- **Flexibility:** The material selected for encapsulation has to provide a proper level of flexibility. Having a flexible package makes the system

bendable and therefore provides better adaptability to the body anatomy. However, the degree of flexibility has to be balanced with the level of support that the package has to provide to the internal electronic circuits to avoid damaging some integrated circuits bonding points or traces. As well, for applications such as pressure measurement, the packaging has to be able to transfer the external pressure to the sensing elements surface.

- **Moisture protection:** The body is an aqueous environment with ions dissolved on it, the ingress of these elements to the internals of an IMS causes failure of the electronic components [108] that can result in harm of the human body. Moisture penetration is one of the most common problems on modern, flexible packaging materials, and the damage resulting from it is irreversible. As well, the moisture absorption on some packaging materials represents a large drift source in pressure sensing systems [109]. The protection against moisture relies in hermeticity, impermeability and adhesion [103].
- **Sterilisation capacity:** Any implantable device has to undergo a systematic, reproducible and validated process for the destruction of any pathogen residing in or on it [7]. This removal of pathogenic and non-pathogenic organisms is defined as sterilisation. This stringent process is designed to destroy the most resistant bacteria spores so that it is ensured that any other element is destroyed. Sterilisation, given its destructive nature, have the potential of damaging or altering the materials that are subjected to the procedure. Given the importance of this process, such materials used for encapsulation must withstand it without significant loss of their performance and characteristics [104]. There are different validated methods for sterilisation; the selection can be made based on the application and materials used in the medical device. In this way, the designer has some room to decide which method is more convenient for the IMS. Some of these methods are [110]:
  - Heat Sterilisation
  - Gaseous Sterilisation
  - Gas Plasma Sterilisation
  - Filtration Sterilisation

6.1.1.2 Available bio-materials

Materials science has provided with several options that can be used in medical devices. As with any design parameter, the material set that can be used depends on the application, expected life-time of the device as well with the environment where it has to operate. The different materials used in medical devices can be classified into two broad categories, hard and soft materials.

Metals, ceramics and glasses compose the hard bio-materials type. Metal bio-materials have been used extensible for the manufacturing of medical implants; they offer high mechanical strength while providing reliable performance in the long-term. Among metal materials used in medical devices is stainless steel, titanium, cobalt alloys, zirconium, tantalum and platinum [105]. In the case of ceramics and glasses, they are known to have high hardness and resistance to wear and corrosion, as well these materials exhibit low conductivity of electricity and heat. However, it is not until recently that modern manufacturing processes are making it possible for these materials to be used more extensively in medical applications [105].

In the other hand, soft bio-materials are composed of biocompatible polymers. These materials, as well as newer moulding, manufacturing and packing techniques, have led to innovation in the area of medical devices and equipment [111]. Concerning medical applications, these materials are interesting for their excellent corrosion resistance, electrical insulation and flexibility. However, permeability and hermeticity are possible sources of problems for implantable devices. Nevertheless, these issues can be attacked by using additives and improving the adhesion of the polymer to the device surface [112]. These materials have attracted the attention of researchers and producers of miniaturised implantable systems. Some common polymers used in medical applications are [111]:

- Polyethylene
- Polypropylene
- Polystyrene
- Polylactic acid
- Polycarbonate
- Polyvinyl Chloride
- Polyethersulfone
- Polyacrylate
- Hydrogels
- Polysulfone
- Polyetheretherketone
- Poly-p-xylylene
- Fluoropolymers
- polysiloxane

6.1.1.3 Encapsulation material selection

The requirements described in Section 6.1.1.1 provide a selection guide of a suitable material for the encapsulation of an IMS. The selection, therefore, depends on the analysis of the specific requirements of the device under development. For the present work, the selected material has to offer the following characteristics:

- High flexibility: The encapsulation has to be flexible and elastic to reduce the risk of fractures by allowing the adaptation of the implant to different anatomies.
- Non-compressible: One of the goals of the implantable device developed in this work is to measure pressure. A non-compressible (and flexible) material allows proper transfer of pressure from the surface of the implantable device to the transducer sensing elements.
- Hermeticity and permeability: The material used has to provide high resistance to moisture absorption, not just to protect the electronic devices, but also to prevent drift on the pressure measurement [12].
- Long term stability: The IMS is expected to survive for long periods when used in human patients since physicians would prefer to avoid a new surgery to remove the device once a therapy has finished. However, for research purposes, a life span of one month is sufficient.

The scope of the present work is restricted to research, and consequently, a limited life-span for the implantable device is acceptable. Also, a commercially available and easy to apply material is preferred (e.g. does not require expensive equipment or highly skilled technicians). Given this reasoning, the conjunction of two materials was chosen for the packaging of the implantable devices: medical-grade silicone (polysiloxane) rubber and parylene-C (Poly-p-xylylene).

Silicone, widely used material for the last 65 years, was chosen to form a base layer for the encapsulation [111]. Silicones are polymeric thermoset elastomers (thermoset). These polymers differentiate from others on the presence of silicon instead of carbon along the main chain [104]. The use of silicone provides advantages as high flexibility, low surface tension, relatively low water absorption and extended mechanical properties stability in a wide temperature range. Furthermore, these materials offer good bio-compatibility. The use of silicone for conformal coatings allows for fast curing cycles with large application yield. As well, for industrial mass applications, the cost per application is low when compared to other coatings in the market [113]. In the medical field, as described in Section 6.1.1.1, sterilisation is a must before the implantation of any device inside a living being. In the case of silicone several methodologies can be used, including dry heat, steam, and radiation techniques [111].

As mentioned, apart of silicone, parylene-C was also selected for the encapsulation of the implantable device. Parylene is the commercial name for Poly-p-xylylenes [103]. Parylene-C (Poly-chloro-para-xylylene) is a variant that includes a chlorine atom on the main chain. This flexible and bio-compatible material provides a much lower water absorption ratio than silicone, making it excellent to be used as an external layer to optimise the hermeticity of a device [12, 112, 114].

The parylene-C coating process is done in three phases [106, 111, 115, 116]. In the first phase, the dichloro-di-p-xylylene dimer is vaporised (at temperatures around 75 °C and 175 °C). In the second phase, the vapour is pyrolysed so that the monomer gas temperature is in the range 650 °C to 700 °C. These two phases are done in a low pressure (lower than 0.6 mbar) chamber. For the third phase, the gaseous monomer is evacuated to a second chamber where the implantable devices are located that is at a lower pressure than the first one and room temperature. In this deposition chamber, the gas is dispersed and spontaneously polymerised on the devices. The coating film produced by this technique can be as thin as few nanometres to as thick as multiple millimetres. Furthermore, the coating produces a uniform encapsulation layer on all sides of the object [111]. The encapsulating layer thickness control, its uniformity and that the devices are not exposed to high temperatures (the IMS remain at room temperature in the deposition chamber) make this process ideal for miniaturised implantable units.

6.1.2 Encapsulation of the pressure monitoring IMS

As mentioned in previous sections, it was decided that the encapsulation for the IMS is designed as a multi-layer process. In the first phase, a layer made of medical-grade silicone [117] has to be applied directly to the electronic board of the device. Then a thin coating of parylene-C is applied to act as a hyper-hydrophobic external protection for the IMS. In the case of the silicone encapsulation, this is done *in-house* using a custom-designed process. In contrast, the most external parylene-C coating was relegated to be done by a third party company using one of their commercially available processes.

The following paragraphs describe the encapsulation of an IMS prototype. First, some considerations for the process flow are presented, followed by the design of the casting mould for silicone and the selection of a separation material. After these subsections, the material preparation and potting processes are described. Finally, some results of the encapsulation are presented.

6.1.2.1 Encapsulation process considerations

After defining the materials to be used in the packaging, a methodical and reproducible encapsulation process has to be defined. A generic workflow for a packaging process has to account at least for the following steps [118]:

- **Cleaning:** A rigorous cleansing process has to be applied to the surface of the object to be coated. This initial step is essential for getting an excellent long-term performance of the encapsulation. Impurities such as solder flux, oils, salts and other particles lead to poor adhesion between the object and the encapsulation material, corrosion, and electrical failures. Salt residues can be easily cleaned with water while oils and fats are removed by using organic solvents and alkaline cleaners.

- **Surface preparation:** With a spotless surface on the device, it needs to be prepared for the coating. The preparation includes a thorough drying procedure to remove any residual water or solvent used during the cleaning. Parts that have been exposed to aqueous solutions might absorb moisture, which then leads to poor adhesion of the encapsulation and bubble formation. The drying is performed by heating the device in an oven (at around 95 °C) for several hours. Moreover, an optional final step on the surface preparation is the application of a primer, which is required when the adhesion between the encapsulation material and the device surface would be otherwise poor.

- **Coating preparation:** The complexity of this step depends on the material chosen for encapsulation. At the end of this stage, the material is ready to be applied to the device.

- **Coating application:** The encapsulation technique selection depends on the application requirements, packaging material, encapsulation reliability, among other factors related to mass production of the implantable device [119]. Different methods are available in order to apply the encapsulation material to an electronic device [118, 119]:

  - Spraying
  - Dipping
  - Molding
  - Glob-topping
  - Potting

- **Dying and curing:** Once the encapsulation material has been applied, it requires curing in order to harden it. This hardening, also known as curing or cross-linking (in polymers), is the process that transforms the material from a soft and liquid form into a hardened one [119]. Each material has to undergo a different procedure in order to cure or polymerise. The most frequent method for epoxies, silicones and other polymers is heat curing. However, other methods such as ultraviolet light polymerisation, and moisture curing are becoming popular since they offer shorter processing times with reduced energy usage and lower volatile emissions [118].
- **Inspection:** For miniaturised electronic devices such as IMS, the applied coatings are thin and therefore, it is difficult to determine their uniformity and if there are areas with insufficient coating [118]. UV indicators or non-destructive thickness measurements can be used to assess any defect in the coating.

The previous flow has to be iterated on multi-layer processes. The complexity and time required per each step depends on the compounds selected on each layer, and some extra steps might be added. When making use of materials that produce a conformal coverage, such as parylene, masking, and de-masking steps have to be added in order to cover parts that are not required to be coated. Furthermore, at the end of a packaging cycle, a designer/manufacturer might weight to rework or discard the devices with faulty packaging. Typically the option is to dispose of the defective units, yet for high-end electronic devices, the relationship gain-effort/cost can outweigh towards reworking the IMS package. However, such decision has to take into account the nature of the materials used in the packaging. As per example, fixing physical defects on encapsulations made of silicone is difficult (due to their low surface free energy) [104], and it can lead to future sources of moisture leakage and degradation of the hermetic seal of the unit. Therefore for a silicone case, an option is to scrape the packaging with a subsequent test of the electronics to make sure that no damage to them has been done. The removal of the damaged encapsulation is done via chemical and mechanical procedures [119]. Parylene, polyimides and epoxies represent the most difficult materials to remove, for these type of coatings, high temperatures, laser ablation or plasma etching processes are required for their removal.

6.1.2.2 Mould design for silicone casting

The casting mould for encapsulating the tumour implant is designed as the negative version of the ideal encapsulation. The mould has to be designed so that the implant can be placed with zero effort in order to limit possible damages to the circuit board. Several options were tested to get the final mould for the production of the prototypes of the implantable device. The list of options tested for the casting mould production are as follows:

- **Additive manufactured mould:** The first trial of a mould for the casting of the silicone encapsulation was done by using additive manufacturing. In this procedure, first, a 3D model of the implantable device was designed. This model was based on the final dimensions and placement of the electronic components. Then, on the same model, the expected encapsulation layer was added. This model is shown in Figure 6.2.a. With this *positive* model, the mould can be designed. As the material available for production was rigid (*clear v4* [120]), the mould was split into six modules that can be easily detached and therefore reduce the stress on the device at the moment of removing it from the mould. The 3D model of the partitioned mould is shown in Figure 6.2.b.

  The mould was fabricated and tested, a sample after some packaging cycles is shown in Figure 6.2.c. The yield of the manufactured parts was low when using this mould. The material used did not support the temperatures required for curing the medical-grade silicone; therefore it became brittle, and after the first cycle it starts shattering (the image shows some of the damages on the mould). However, this method provided an economical and fast way to test the encapsulation process and to fine-tune the package dimensions. The original *positive* model was useful as well for the next methods.

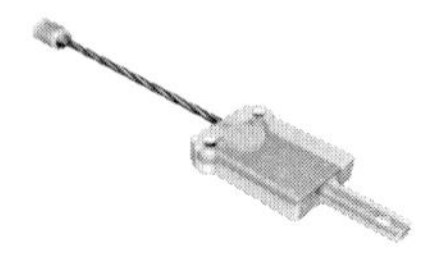

(a) 3D model for tumour monitoring implant used for the mould design (including expected silicone encapsulation).

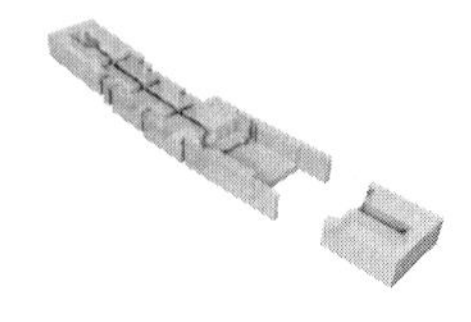

(b) 3D model for manufacturing the mould.

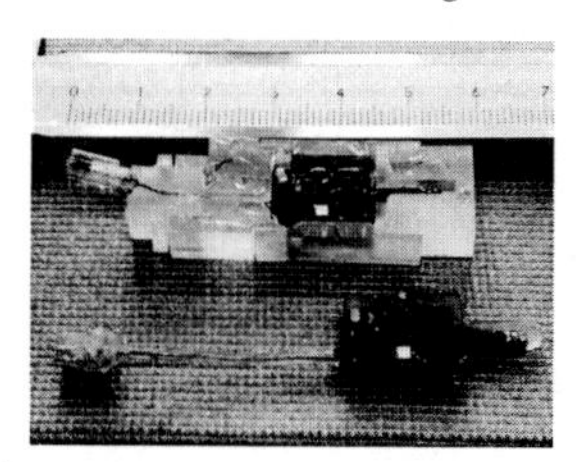

(c) Mould sample and a packaged IMS.

FIGURE 6.2: Mould produced using additive manufacturing.

- **Silicone mould:** For the fabrication of this mould, a two component-silicone rubber was chosen [121]. This material can withstand temperatures up to 230 °C. For the production of the mould, a *positive* of the implantable device was designed, as shown in Figure 6.3. Some extra chambers were added to allow flow of extra silicone to the sides.

  After preparing the material for the mould, it was poured in a rectangular container, and then the *positive* of the implantable device was placed on top. A commercially available sprayed release agent [122] was used between the 3D printed template and the silicone. After curing and inspecting the part, and without removing the *positive*, a release agent layer was applied to the top of the fabricated part. Then, silicone was poured on top and placed in the oven for curing. The result was the two parts silicone mould. Thanks to the release agent applied, the two pieces were able to get separated (from each other and the template).

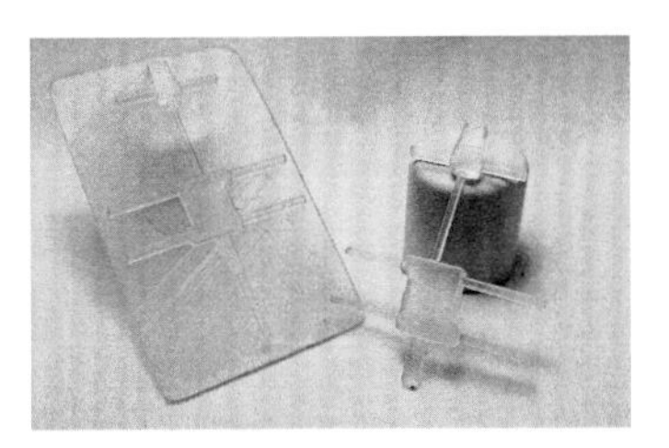

FIGURE 6.3: 3D model of the *Positive* for silicone-made mould fabrication (based on the design in Figure 6.2.a).

With this new mould, a packaging test, using a mock-up part, was performed. The same release agent [122] was sprayed to the mould making sure to have a uniform layer. The medical-grade silicone was prepared and poured in the bottom part of the mould. Afterwards, the implant was placed on the mould, and more silicone poured. Finally, the top part of the mould was placed on top and pressed. This arrangement of parts was placed in the oven for the silicone to be cured. At the end of the curing process, the part was removed from the mould, yet problems such as material leaking through the mould sides, and damages to the test IMS happened. Due to this problems, the silicone mould was not used, and a third option was designed.

- **Machined mould in Polytetrafluoroethylene (PTFE):** After the experience with the moulds in silicone and additive manufactured, the final option was to use PTFE as the material for the mould. Even when this material is not flexible, it offers low adhesion to the silicone used as packaging. In the case of this mould, it was machined directly from a CAD file. The design is based on the same *positive* model in Figure 6.3, but the CAD file contains a *negative* version of it. Apart from the space for the implant and the silicone, two guides were added to improve alignment. The resulting mould is shown in Figure 6.4.a, while a part fabricated with this version is shown in Figure 6.4.b.

  As appreciated in Figure 6.4.a, the mould was able to withstand several encapsulation cycles without altering its mechanical properties. In order to reduce *flash* [123], the mould was pressed tightly with clamps during curing. Sprayed release agent [122] was used as an extra precaution to avoid the encapsulation to stick to the mould. Figure 6.4.b shows an implant successfully encapsulated using this final mould.

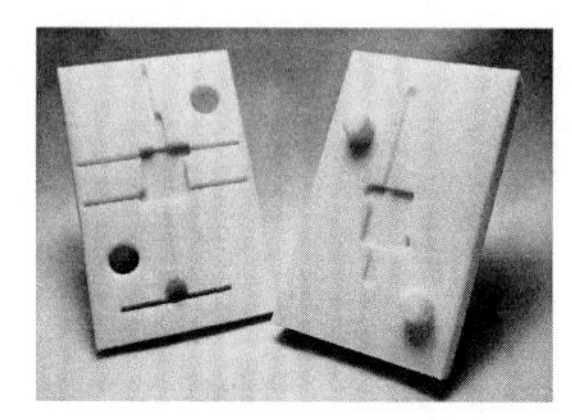

(a) PTFE-made mould after several encapsulation cycles.

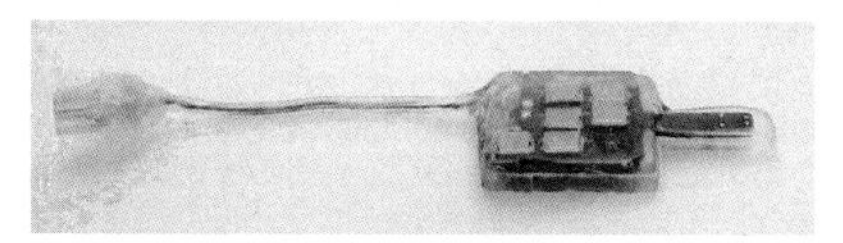

(b) Packaged IMS using the Teflon-mould.

FIGURE 6.4: Mould produced using PTFE.

6.1.2.3 Silicone preparation and potting

As described in Section 6.1.1.3, the first coating for the IMS is made of medical-grade silicone. A commercially available two-parts silicone was chosen [117]. The first step for the preparation of the material was to remove any air bubbles from the two parts used in this silicone. For this purpose, a vacuum chamber was used. Since the application was made with a manual dispenser/mixer, each part was poured on a separate chamber before degassing.

A primer [124] was applied to the electronic board to strengthen the adhesion of the silicone to the implantable device surface. The application of the primer was made manually with a brush. In the other hand, a release agent [122] was applied to both parts of the PTFE mould to reduce adhesion between the encapsulation and mould.

Finally, the degassed silicone parts were applied (and mixed at the same time) to the PTFE mould and the electronic device. Then the mould was tightly closed using clamps to reduce the chance of *flash* [123]. For the material curing process, the mould with the silicone and IMS was placed in an oven at 150 °C for 15 minutes. The result of this encapsulation process is shown in Figure 6.4.b.

The packaged implants were able to work during in-vivo experiments. The dual coating process protected the electronics from fluids, as well allowed to correctly measure the pressure and temperature of a tumour (as described in Section 7.2.5).

6.2 Manufacturing of mechanical parts [125]

As described in Section 2.1, IMS small dimensions are a design challenge, which affects not only the decisions regarding electronic components but also the selection of mechanical parts required. It is possible to find *off-the-shelf* mechanical elements, such as connectors and fittings. However, most of the time, using these commercially available parts results in compromises on the possible materials, geometry and features. Moreover, some parts might not be available in small quantities (as needed for prototyping).

An alternative, to avoid compromising the IMS design, is to request custom made parts from an external manufacturer. However, this type of service is not always available, and if so it usually means a high cost for small quantities (e.g., the initial costs of producing a custom part). The last argument is not valid for mass production purposes, where the cost per part would decrease with large volumes.

In the case of this work, whose purpose is to produce the prototypes of an IMS, buying external parts or requesting custom elements are no options. Therefore, the use of additive manufacturing was the best option for getting the required mechanical elements.

One requirement for the prototype prepared in this work (Described in detail in Chapter 7) was to develop a wired connection between the IMS and the reader-hardware. The physical implementation of this interface needed small connectors and a support to fix them on the test-mice during animal experiments. For this purpose, a set of parts was design and fabricated using additive manufacturing. Figure 6.5 shows a 3D rendering and a photograph of the manufactured parts.

In the case of the IMS connector, it has four holes for holding female contacts with an external diameter of 0.9 mm. Furthermore, the connector has three guides on its side to ensure the pin-order when used together with the port and reader adapter. The total radius of the connector is 3 mm (without including the guides to the sides).

After deployed of the IMS inside the test mouse, its connector remains outside the animal body. The port (annotated as 3 in Figure 6.5), is used to fix this connector to the animal skin. Once the connector has been inserted on the port, the surgeon sutures this last part in the mouse skin using several holes provided on it (at the bottom of the port). A tiny screw (on the side of

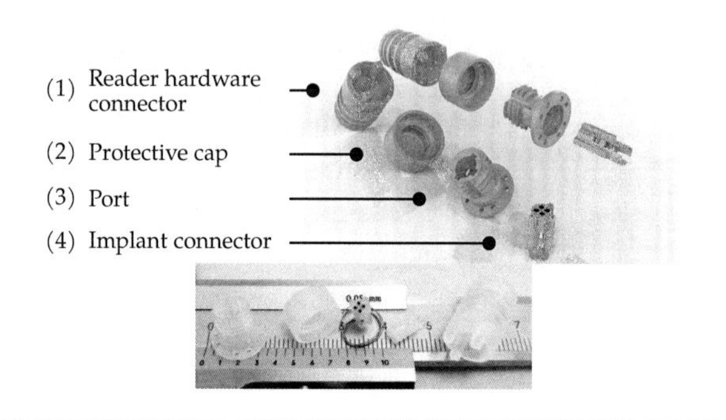

FIGURE 6.5: Custom mechanical parts fabricated using additive manufacturing (metal pins added for illustration). Top: 3D rendering, Bottom: Photograph of fabricated parts.

the port) secures the connector port structure. Finally, a cap can be screwed to the port to protect it against fluids or other external agents (annotated as 2 in Figure 6.5).

The final part required was an adapter to connect the reader-hardware to the implant. Figure 6.5 shows the developed part annotated as 1. This part includes four holes with a 1 mm diameter to hold the male pins used to contact the IMS (the pin contact part is 0.45 mm). This adapter has three guides that match three slots in the port element, which ensures the proper pin order when connecting.

The mentioned parts were manufactured using Stereolithography and a *clear* resin material [120]. This material is not graded as bio-compatible [126]; therefore, the parts were coated with a layer of medical-grade silicone [117] and parylene-C. The application of this coating treatment ensured the safety of the tissues in contact with the IMS surfaces.

6.3 Manufacture of mockups

The development of medical systems requires the interaction of engineers (from electronics, material science, among others) and physicians. The exchange of expertise between these fields is critical in the first design phases of a medical system. From this interaction allows the definition of the electrical and mechanical specifications for the design. Furthermore, the fabrication of phantom systems allow engineers to evaluate IMS before any in-vivo test [127].

Regarding the mechanical specifications, the human body geometry represents a challenge. The implantation location, depth, surrounding tissue properties, as well as if there is much movement or not, result on constraints for the IMS geometry and mechanical characteristics (e.g., flexibility). These properties that affect the IMS mechanical specifications are well known to physicians, and therefore their input on this topic is essential for a successful project completion.

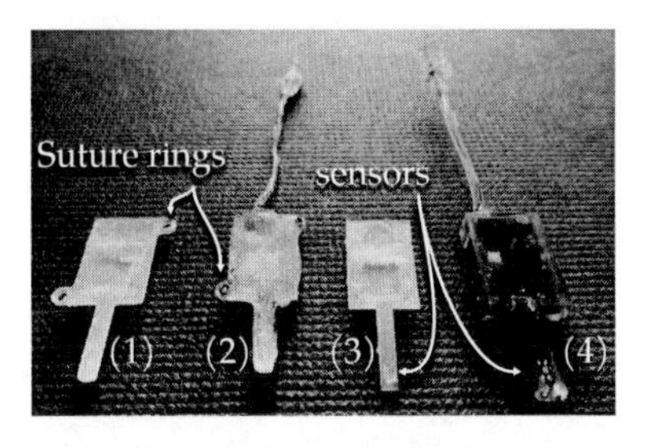

FIGURE 6.6: Some of the 3D printed mechanical prototypes of the IMS. 1. First version of the IMS with suturing rings included, 2. A prototype *packaged* in silicone for implantation procedure practice, 3. Final version of the IMS, 4. Real packaged IMS (for comparison purposes).

In this work, a practical solution for the definition of these mechanical specifications was to use additively manufactured prototypes. These prototypes were designed in a CAD software based on an initial input from the physicians, as well from the geometry of the electronic components used. These prototypes were provided to the physicians to verify the dimensions of the IMS mainboard, wires, and connectors. Furthermore, a layer of silicone was applied to some prototypes so that they could be used to practice the implantation procedure (on already dead mice).

Figure 6.6 shows some of the developed prototypes together with the final version of the IMS. The use of these prototypes helped to get mechanical specifications that did not change during the presented work. Moreover, having these robust mechanical definitions was essential for the documentation needed to get the experiments approval from an animal ethical committee.

Chapter 7

Application in cancer monitoring

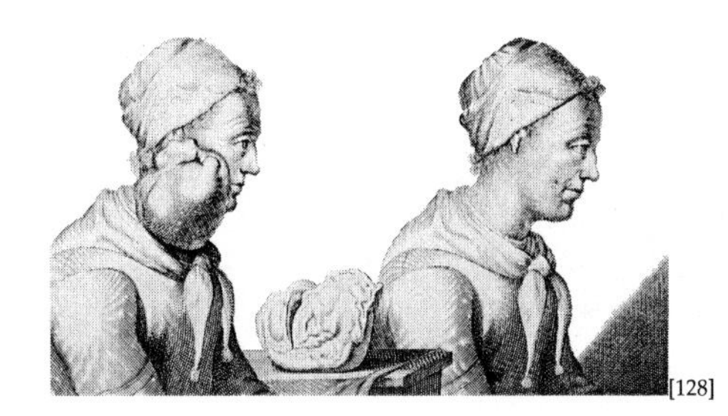

[128]

Greek physician and philosopher Hippocrates (460-370 BC), known as "Father of Medicine", was the first to use the term *karkinos* to refer to what we know as cancer nowadays. Historians believe that the chosen word reflects the tenacity of these lesions, their high recurrence rate, and their ability to spread to distant places in the body. The earliest references (in the western hemisphere) to this disease was found in Egyptian papyrus dating to around 1500 BC [129]. By 2012, cancer have accounted for approximately 14 million cases, as well as 8 million deaths around the globe. Furthermore, there is an estimated (2012) of 165 thousand cases of cancer in children (up to 14 years old) [130]. It is only expected for these numbers to grow because the global population is more exposed to factors that favour the development of cancer such as obesity, tobacco use, pollution, and pathogens as the papillomavirus.

It was not until the last century that the most critical milestones in cancer research and treatment were achieved. The 19th century saw the invention of the microscope, which gave scientists new insights about the cell, as well as the invention of X-rays, which gave birth to radiology. Furthermore, in the post-Second-World-War era, the research on radioactivity led to what now is known as nuclear medicine and the later invention of computer tomography.

Together with better tools to diagnose cancer, newer ways to attack this disease have also been conceived in the last century. For instance, during the Second World War, research on the military applications of mustard gas led to the finding of a compound called nitrogen mustard, which worked against lymphomas. This discovery served to ignite interest in the research and development of compounds that targeted the DNA of cancerous cells [129]. Besides chemotherapy, which is still the main line of treatment for cancer, other techniques such as Hormone therapy and immunotherapy have been developed in the last decades. However, a need exists for suitable biomarkers that can provide insight into the effectiveness and response ratios for such therapies and thus improving the overall survival ratio [131].

This chapter presents the use of two biomarkers to monitor the status of a tumour: interstitial fluid pressure and temperature. The first part describes the cancer micro-environment and how the measured parameters are related to its evolution. With this theory, the second part describes the design of an implantable system prototype for the measurement of temperature and pressure in a tumour. Finally, results from in-vivo tests are presented which prove the concept developed in this work.

7.1 Cancer and its micro-environment

For decades, the focus of cancer research was on the cancerous cells internal mechanisms and the way its genetics get altered. However, nowadays, researchers are looking outside these cells and finding that tumours behave as multicellular organisms and that the key for its cure might be on the surroundings of cancerous cells [132]. As described in Section 2.2, in a healthy individual, the interstitial and the micro-circulatory system allows for the delivery of the components (nutrients, minerals, oxygen, drugs, among others) required for the correct functions of the different tissues, as well as routing the waste materials to the bloodstream for its subsequent disposal.

This interstitial space exists surrounded by the stroma (microenvironment). Cells such as fibroblasts, epithelial, inflammatory, immunocytes, and vascular [133], among others forms the stroma. Additionally, the Extracellular Matrix (ECM) is part of the stroma. This network (the ECM) is composed of macromolecules such as collagen, glycoproteins, and enzymes. Under normal conditions, the ECM has a structural support function by providing a three-dimensional substrate to where cells adhere. Furthermore, the ECM brings guidance for the alignment and direction of tissue growth; as well as assisting on the intercellular signal transfer [134].

Researchers have identified that during the process of carcinogenesis, the tumorous cells alter the balance in the interstitial space. These alterations promote a microenvironment that amplifies the tumour growth [18]. The cancer tissue triggers a set of pathways that form positive feedback loops between the different characteristics of the interstitial space; some of these interactions are shown in the flow diagram in Figure 7.1. The evolution monitoring of these microenvironment properties provides to physicians and researches novel biomarkers. The continuous evaluation of these biomarkers leads to an improved understanding of the status of a given tumour and therefore, asses a better prognosis of the applied therapeutics [136]. From all these possible biomarkers, this work focuses on the Interstitial Fluid Pressure (IFP) monitoring.

7.1.1 Role of interstitial fluid pressure in cancer development and treatment

During its initial phases, a tumour takes nutrients and oxygen from the bloodstream, through the normal processes described in Section 2.2. At some point, the local vascular system (and the flow of nutrients and gases) becomes

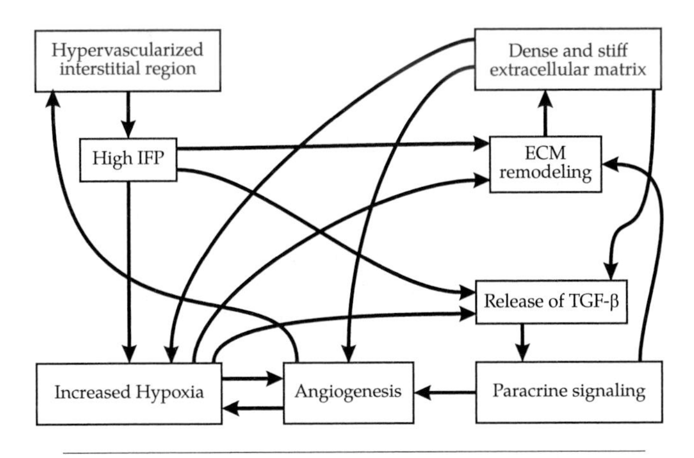

FIGURE 7.1: Relation between biological processes and characteristics that promote the micro-environment of a tumour (adapted from [135]).

insufficient due to the continuous growth of the tumour [137]. This deficiency produces a reduction on the available oxygen for the cancerous cells, which results in a hypoxic environment that triggers the various vicious cycles shown in Figure 7.1, such as excessive angiogenesis, release of Transforming Growth Factor Beta (TGF-β) and ECM remodelling [131, 137, 138].

7.1.1.1 Overview of the tumour micro-environment development

After the establishment of cancerous cells in an organ, they start multiplying thanks to the nutrients provided by the host micro-circulatory system. As previously explained, there is a point where the normal vascular system becomes insufficient to sustain the uncontrolled growth of the tumour. As well, as shown in Figure 7.1, the same tumour stroma (dense and stiff extracellular matrix) can cause further obstruction of the vessels and therefore worsening the whole shortage of nutrients and oxygen [16]. This process then leads to hypoxia.

As described, hypoxia (a general feature in solid tumours) is a critical characteristic that amplifies the aggressiveness of tumours and worsens the genomic stability [138]. Hypoxic conditions are highly toxic for cancerous cells, as with normal tissue. However, several genetic changes allow the tumour cells to proliferate in these conditions, and instead been destroyed, amplifies the tumour malignancy and aggressiveness. Parts of these adaptations are the metabolic reprogramming mediated by Hypoxia-inducible factor–1α (HIF-1 α), activated under these hypoxic conditions [137, 139].

The activation of HIF-1 α in conjunction with Vascular Endothelial Growth Factor (VEGF) triggers tumour-induced angiogenesis [137, 140]. This process creates new but imperfect blood vessels to supply the demands of oxygen and nutrients from the growing tumour. The developed vascular network presents leaky and irregular vessels [16]. The constant presence of Vascular Endothelial Growth Factor (VEGF) causes the leak of plasma fibrinogen which induces the excessive creation and spread of new vessels in the tumour area [139].

The leakiness of the newly formed and imperfect vascular network, together with the lack of lymphatic vessels produces a constant flow of fluid into the interstitial space and therefore an abnormal increment of the interstitial fluid pressure. As the IFP increases, it reaches a point where it reaches a value p_0 that causes, by the Starling law (Equation 2.2), a pressure barrier for the fluid flux. The consequence is the formation of a necrotic core [19], as shown in the simplified model in Figure 7.2. Chronic hypoxia is present in this area since no functional vessels are present [138].

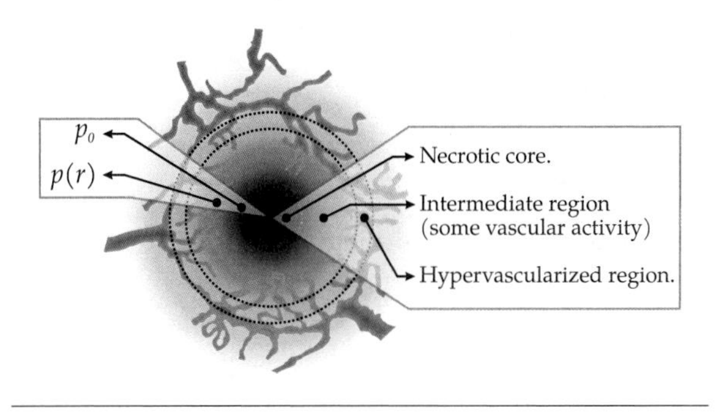

FIGURE 7.2: Simplified model of tumour structure (based on [19]).

Tumour cells outside the necrotic core experience acute hypoxia mainly due to temporal vessel occlusion (the tumour vascular system is fragile) and the relative high IFP. The pressure presents a decreasing value towards the limits of the tumour. As illustrated in Figure 7.2, the hyper-vascularised region in the outer part of the tumour presents the lower pressure providing with the required nutrients and oxygen to the most external cancerous cells. As the tumour grows, this vicious cycle continues, with the creation of ad blood vessels and the increase of the IFP [16].

As described in Section 2.2, under normal conditions, the hydrostatic interstitial fluid pressure has values in the range -1 mmHg to -3 mmHg [16]. However, due to the described processes, the IFP in tumours is around 10 mmHg to 30 mmHg higher than in healthy tissue, and values as high as 60 mmHg have been observed [141].

7.1.1.2 Tumour micro-environment effects on cancer treatment

As previously described, the permissive microenvironment developed during carcinogenesis (which for normal tissue would be considered adverse) provides the perfect components for the uncontrolled growth of the tumour. Moreover, this microenvironment establishes the conditions needed for the natural selection of the most aggressive clones and further metastasis [19, 137]. However, the benefit that this aggressive microenvironment provides to the tumour development goes further and acts as a protection against therapy.

The significantly large (compared to healthy tissue) osmotic and hydrostatic pressure present in a tumour (as previously presented), creates a barrier to the transport of therapeutic agents into the tumours. This effect on the intake of therapeutic elements is a direct consequence of a restricted fluid flux into the tumour. This reduced flow is the product of several factors of Starling law (Equation 2.2) outside their normal ranges due to the tumorous microenvironment [17].

In the case of chemotherapy and immunotherapy, the reduced flow due to the increased interstitial pressure leads to a decreased acceptance of drugs or antibodies into the tumour. This reduced uptake limits the concentration of agents inside the tumour, and therefore the therapy efficiency is lowered [16]. Similarly, it has been reported that the tumour stroma influences negatively modern cancer nano-therapeutics efficiency. Even when the high permeability of the defective tumour vascular network can be advantageous for the intratumoral delivery of the nano-therapeutics, the large IFP limits the access of these agents to hyper-vascularised region [142].

Radiotherapy is also indirectly affected by the elevated IFP through hypoxia. Some studies propose that the increased hypoxic environment found in the interior of the tumour, due to the increased interstitial pressure values, is related to radioresistance causing a decrease in the overall therapy effectiveness [138, 143].

The recognition of the role played by the microenvironment on the tumour aggressiveness, and resistance to treatment is a milestone in cancer research. This concept has led researchers to find ways of reducing the microenvironment's influence via new or complementary therapies [144]. One of the techniques used to reduce the effects of the microenvironment on therapy is the application of heat to the tumour area, known as hyperthermia [145]. In this technique, the application of heat to a specific region of the body triggers different biological reactions aimed at restoring the normal temperature. The body's reaction to heat alters the tumour microenvironment as well improves the immune response [145]. During localised hyperthermia, target temperatures in the range 42 °C to 45 °C induce cytotoxicity, thus causing the death of cancerous cells as well as the destruction of tumour vascular endothelium [143]. Furthermore, research has found that moderate temperature increase (39 °C to 42 °C) is also beneficial since it provides radiosensitisation by improving oxygenation and vascular perfusion [143].

The use of antiangiogenic drugs is another technique being explored that aims to disrupt the tumour microenvironment. As previously described, angiogenesis is a critical element for the development of an aggressive microenvironment (Figure 7.1); therefore, a good target for therapy. The application of these drugs promotes the tumour absorption of medications as well as improves the efficiency of radiotherapy [146]. This technique also can help to kill cancerous cells by starving them (reduced nutrients and oxygen due to limited angiogenesis) [132].

These well-known techniques (e.g., hyperthermia), as well as experimental ones (e.g., ultrasound and microbubbles targeted on direct IFP reduction [147]) that attack the tumour microenvironment, show promise in helping physicians to improve tumour treatments.

7.1.2 Importance of tumour interstitial fluid pressure monitoring

A critical problem to solve for therapies targeting the microenvironment is to assess their efficacy and to quantise their effect. Furthermore, some of these therapies are only effective within a small *window of opportunity*. For instance, in the case of using anti-angiogenesis drugs, the right amount helps to reduce the vascular capacity of the tumour to typical values. However, excess of these agents results in hypo-vascularisation and therefore limiting the access of chemotherapy agents into the tumour [146]. Furthermore, the hypoxia that is produced by excessive reduction of the vascular capacity can produce, over time, resistance to these agents [132, 137]. The obstacles mentioned above call for improved monitoring of tumour microenvironment status.

Furthermore, an improved monitoring and evaluation of biomarkers in the tumour microenvironment could allow for better diagnosis, prognosis and to predict the efficiency of a given therapy (it has been observed that a successful therapy leads to a reduction of IFP [131]). The information extracted from the microenvironment could lead to tailored therapies that take into account individual genetic and metabolic characteristics, as well as the adjustment of such therapies over time, based on the tumour response [136, 141].

As explained, IFP has a high impact on the tumour microenvironment development. The monitoring of IFP specifically has the potential to estimate the tumour evolution (e.g., size, stage) as well as predict its resistance to therapy [131]. Research has also found that techniques such as hyperthermia or antiangiogenic drugs, among others, can induce changes in the IFP via variations on the tumour vascular system [131, 143, 146]. Therefore, physicians would be able to determine the *window of opportunity* for these therapies by having at hand the current value of tumour IFP.

7.1.2.1 Interstitial fluid pressure monitoring methods

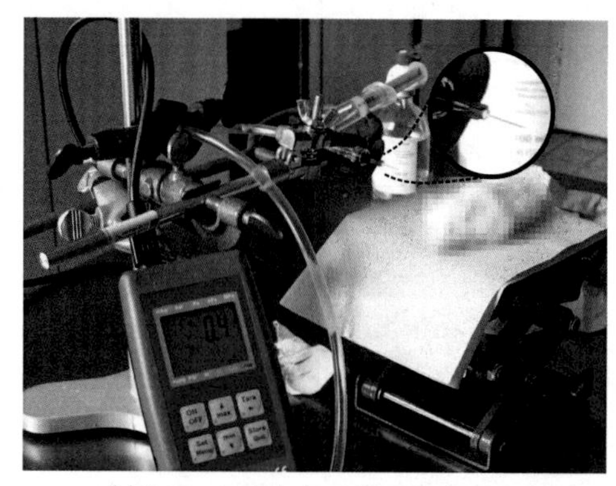

(a) Setup example for mice experiments.

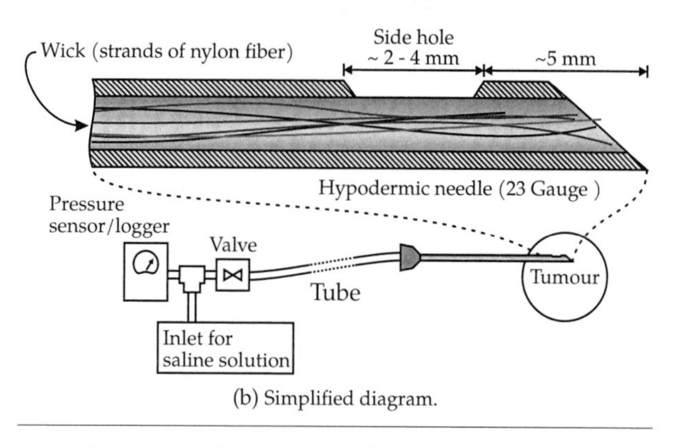

(b) Simplified diagram.

FIGURE 7.3: Wick-in-needle IFP measurement setup.

As described, IFP is a valid biomarker for the diagnosis of cancer and the prognosis of different treatments. This variable, which usually presents a negative value (Section 2.2), has a consistent behaviour during the growth of a tumour (increasing pressure) and when a therapy is effective (decreasing IFP), as described in the previous section.

The first successful measurement of interstitial fluid pressure was taken in 1963 via an implantable capsule proposed by Guyton [148] (who determined that IFP has a small negative value). In 1968, Scholander introduced the wick catheter technique [149], which was later improved by Fadnes in 1977 with his Wick-in-Needle technique [150]. Unfortunately, these techniques require surgery as well as complex instrumentation setups.

The Wick-in-Needle technique is still commonly accepted as the gold standard procedure for IFP measurement [151]. Figure 7.3.a shows the setup for a Wick-in-Needle test on mice. In this setup, a hypodermic needle with a side opening, as presented in Figure 7.3.b, is filled with strands of nylon fibres and tubes connect the needle to a pressure reading interface. Before the measurement, the system is filled with a saline solution, taking care to remove any air bubbles. The needle is then inserted in such a way that the side hole is located in the area of interest (e.g., tumour) [150, 152]. The subject has to be immobilised to avoid artefacts in the measurement, meaning experimental animals have to be fully anaesthetised.

Although the results from the Wick-in-Needle technique are reliable, it is impractical for clinical use. Various non-invasive techniques have been explored over the years. The work in [141] proposed the use of ultrasound equipment together with a mixture of ultrasound contrast agents and gas microbubbles. Likewise, [153, 154] have proven that Magnetic Resonance Imaging (MRI) can be used to determine the fluid flow and interstitial fluid pressure in tumours indirectly.

These IFP measuring methods reduce the risk associated with an invasive technique (e.g., Wick-in-needle). However, the number of MRI or Ultrasound devices in the health care system is small. It, therefore, imposes a limitation on the chances to take measurements from an individual patient during a whole treatment cycle. Additionally, even if the resources would be accessible, taking readings with these devices several times a day becomes impractical for patients as well as for the healthcare professional in charge.

7.1.3 Applications of intratumoral temperature monitoring

As already discussed, the tumour microenvironment represents a complex system where the cancerous cells alter various biological mechanisms. The progression of a tumour and its surrounding stroma induces specific changes in several bio-parameters, including interstitial pressure (presented in Section 7.1.2) and temperature.

Since the 1970s, several studies have shown that temperature readings are useful to diagnose tumours. These first studies focused on breast cancer and used infrared imaging as a measuring method [155]. Usage of thermal images for the study of tumours has shown promising results, and nowadays, some literature is also complementing it with deep learning techniques [156].

The work in [157] reported that when using infrared imaging, breast tumours can be detected on patients thanks to a 1 °C to 2 °C skin temperature increase at their periphery. These results are consistent with measurements done by inserting a micro thermocouple into the tumour [158].

Furthermore, tests on mouse xenografts of breast cancer (MDA-MB-231, MCF7, and 13762 MAT cell lines) found, through thermal imaging, a correlation between the tumour size and reduction in its temperature [157, 159]. The contrast between these results and those found in humans is not well understood, but it is thought that it has to do with the differences between a tumour in a human patient and a xenograft [157]. Nevertheless, both types of studies present compelling evidence to use temperature monitoring as a tool for research and clinical applications on cancer.

Besides its use for diagnosis and prognosis, temperature monitoring could improve current therapies. As presented in Section 7.1.1.2, the use of hyperthermia increases the uptake of therapeutic agents into the tumour. Intratumoral temperature monitoring can help determine when the tumour has reached the optimum temperature. Providing this information to physicians in real-time could limit the heat application to only what is necessary, therefore improving the patient's comfort and reducing any side effects.

7.2 Implantable medical system for cancer monitoring

The previous chapters have been devoted to the description of the minimum blocks required in the datapath of an implantable system for invasive pressure monitoring. Furthermore, a timing unit for such a low data rate system was proposed. These blocks provide the foundation for a fully functional and low power implantable device for pressure monitoring. Considerations for the encapsulation and prototyping of a device that handles pressure and temperature monitoring were also presented.

In this section, a proof of concept is presented for the temperature and pressure continuous monitoring in cancerous tumours via an IMS. A prototype was implemented and tested to validate the design concepts explored during the present work and to define, based on these results, the further requirements of a system for clinical use.

7.2.1 State of the art

In 1963, Guyton proposed an implantable perforated chamber for IFP measurement. These capsules were implanted in the tissue and left to fill with interstitial fluid for about three weeks. The pressure inside the capsule was monitored via a small needle inserted (through the skin) into one of the capsule's perforations [148]. With this method, Guyton was able to determine the value of IFP in several experiments. This technique provides better results than the wick-in-needle since it overcomes possible problems from the use of needles whose diameter was larger than the interstitial space, however at the price of a more complex procedure.

In 2016, Seung Song proposed the use of electronic components to improve the Guyton chamber [146]. The developed device used an L-C based transducer that translated the pressure applied into variations on its resonance frequency. The achieved resolution on this setup was 1 mmHg. The device presents a round geometry with 3 mm of diameter and a thickness of 1 mm.

7.2.2 Implant electronic module

Based on the medical systems categories described in Section 2.1, a device developed for the evaluation of the tumour microenvironment falls into the category of monitoring IMS. As already presented, these devices allow researchers and physicians to access one or several biomarkers from inside the body.

As stated, this research's purpose is to lay the foundation for the successful development of an IMS for cancer monitoring. In these initial steps, a proof-of-concept system was required to explore the feasibility of such devices, as well as to verify the continuous acquisition of information from the tumour. Guided by these concerns, the prototype presented in this section prioritised the core components related to the data path in the general diagram

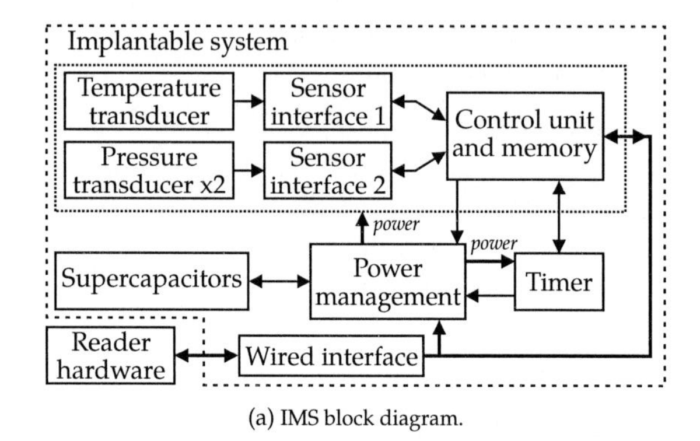

(a) IMS block diagram.

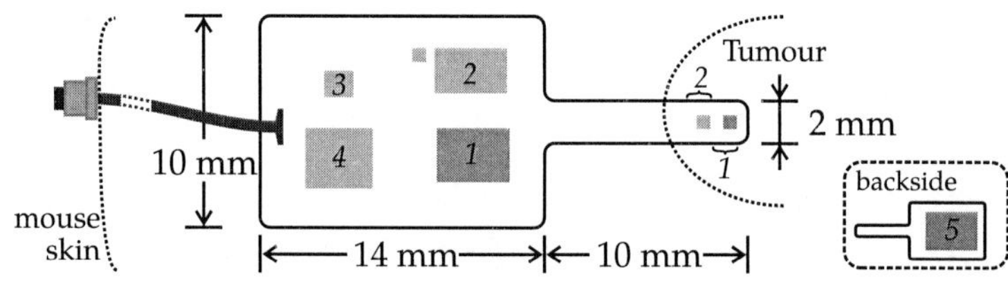

(b) IMS floorplan (not to scale): (1) pressure transducer and its interface, (2) temperature sensors and their interface, (3) timing unit, (4) control unit, power management and memory, (5) super-capacitor bank.

FIGURE 7.4: Block diagram and floorplan for the prototype of cancer monitoring IMS.

in Figure 2.1. For this reason, the wireless energy harvesting and telemetry units are not present in this phase of work and are replaced by a more robust but straightforward wired interface, resulting in the block diagram shown in Figure 7.4.a.

As presented in Figure 7.4.a, the temperature and pressure transducers use separate interfaces; It was thus possible to tailor each path to the characteristics of each sensing element. A control unit together with a timing unit takes care of the signals required to enable or disable the sensing units as well as storing the information retrieved and handling communications. As for power management, a low-power LDO was used; however, for a final implementation, the use of more advanced dc-to-dc converters is recommended [160].

A super-capacitor bank was used as the energy storage unit to provide autonomy to the device. As described in [161], our experiments showed the potential of super-capacitors for implantable systems. By powering low-power IMS with miniature versions of these devices it is possible to obtain long run times while requiring short charging times (e.g., less than one minute). The fast charging is particularly crucial for the prototype discussed in this section. Since a wired connection was implemented, the animals used in the in vivo tests had to be sedated for charging and retrieving data, therefore reducing the time required for such actions was essential to reduce the risks related to general anaesthetics.

As described in Section 6.3, part of the initial design phase was the definition of the mechanical parameters for the IMS. These were obtained through the use of 3D printed prototype models provided to the physicians involved in the proof-of-concept experiments. Following this process, it was possible to define the geometry and floor plan for the implant, which are shown in Figure 7.4.b (the different colours identify each block). As presented in the diagram, a narrow tip is used to locate the pressure and temperature transducers inside the tumour under study. The rest of the blocks presented in Figure 7.4.a are distributed in a more extensive section of the implant.

It is essential to highlight that, as shown in the floorplan, a secondary temperature sensor was added close to the interfaces and outside the tumour area. This transducer provides the tissue temperature outside the tumour, while at the same time allows for determining if the electronics or storage elements overheat when active or under recharge. The readings from the external transducers are used for further characterisation of the temperature dependency of the IMS blocks as well. Similarly, the measurements from the temperature sensor in the measuring tip are also used to compensate the pressure sensor output (described below in Section 7.2.3).

Figure 7.5 shows an annotated photography of the prototype IMS. The device includes the mechanical parts presented in Section 6.2. As described in Section 6.1, the encapsulation of the IMS consisted of a thick layer of medical-grade silicone and a thin layer of parylene-C. The proposed encapsulation provides a robust protection for the electronics and the host while allowing for correct reading of the pressure. The total volume of the sensing tip, as indicated in Figure 7.5, is 10.5 mm $\times$ 3 mm $\times$ 1.6 mm. The medical researchers verified (via the use of 3D printed models) that these dimensions allow the sensors to be placed inside a tumour.

The system state machine has two principal operational modes: Autonomous mode and Controlled mode. A flow diagram representing the state

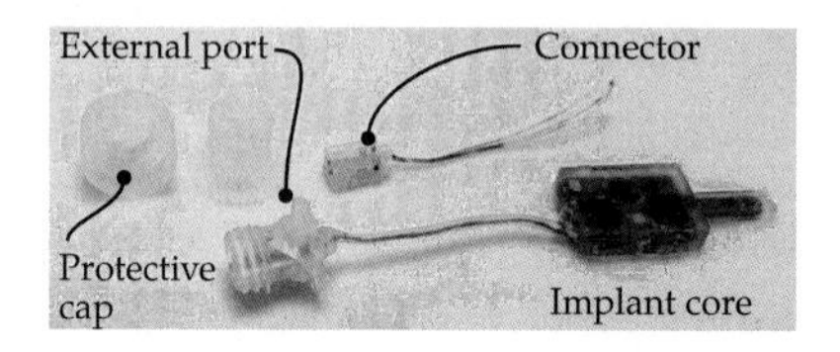

FIGURE 7.5: Annotated photograph of the first implant prototype.

machine that implements the control unit is shown in Figure 7.6. Most of the time, the system remains in an idle state where only the timer unit is powered, and therefore the average system power consumption is in the nanowatt range (Section 5).

During regular operation (autonomous mode), the system is woken up by the output signal from the timer, setting the system to acquire a temperature and pressure sample. During sampling, the IMS first enables the transducers and their interfaces. In subsequent steps, the IMS digitises the data available at the output of each sensor and saves it to memory. It is important to emphasise that the IMS only stores the raw data generated from the sensors and does not apply any processing. By doing so, the IMS saves energy and allows for a system with reduced complexity and area. After storing the pressure and temperature samples, the sensors are disabled, and then the state machine forces the system to go back to the idle state.

During the *active* phase in the autonomous mode (i.e., the process followed after a timer trigger event), the device power consumption reaches its maximum, and therefore it has been optimised for speed. The main contribution to the *active* time is the sampling process, which depends on the sensor stabilisation time as well as the interface characteristics (described in Section 3.2).

The second operational mode (controlled), serves two purposes: first, it allows the recovery of information from the device (database), and the second is to configure the system before a measuring cycle. The device configuration consists of parameters such as sampling time (which is passed to the timer unit) and calibration data (only stored in memory), among others. Additionally, during this mode, it is possible to request the performance of a single measurement to get a sample value of the current pressure and temperature(`Get a single sample`). This last option is useful for the device

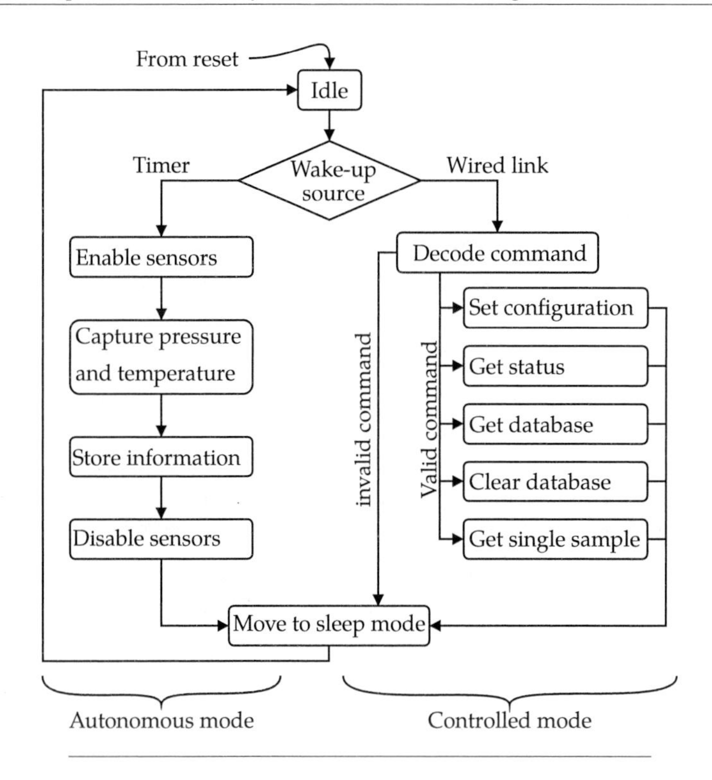

FIGURE 7.6: Flow diagram for the IMS internal state machine.

calibration, debugging, as well to have a *live* measurement setup.

The data recovery commands `Get database` and `Get status` provide the reader hardware with all the samples acquired through the autonomous mode. Furthermore, part of the data provided is the timestamp for the start of the current measurement cycle, as well as the calibration parameters assigned to the IMS. With this data, the reader hardware applies the right compensation to the raw data (as mentioned, the IMS does not apply corrections) so that the user has access to useful information.

It is relevant to indicate that during the controlled mode, the IMS is also charged so that it is prepared for the next measuring cycle. As shown in Figure 7.4, the energy is stored in a bank of miniature super-capacitors.

7.2.3 Sensor Calibration

Medical devices become helpful tools for physicians and researchers only if the information they provide is meaningful. These devices rely on sensors that translate a patient's physical, biochemical, or physiological variables, as well as the environmental variables that surround him/her into electrical signals that are processed electronically. The reliability of the data acquired by these sensors assures the proper operation of the medical instruments so that they can provide essential information for the health professionals decision-making, as well for medical and technological research and development.

Unknown deviations on the measurements provided by medical instruments expose patients to hazardous situations, where therapies are not adjusted properly, and place can even lead to life-threatening situations [162]. Furthermore, hidden errors jeopardise the interpretation of data, leading researchers to wrong conclusions or misleading characterisation of designs.

7.2.3.1 Accuracy and Precision in sensing devices

Two common ways to determine the validity of the information generated by an instrument are through its accuracy and precision. These two parameters are critical parts of any product specification, yet despite their importance, sometimes are confusing parameters on system design. Figure 7.7 provides a graphical interpretation of these two parameters. As seen, the distance between the reference or *true* value is analogue to accuracy, the closer the average device measurement to this reference, the more accurate the instrument is. On the other hand, the probability distribution of the measurements around the average indicates the accuracy of the instrument. Precise sensor systems would provide narrow distributions.

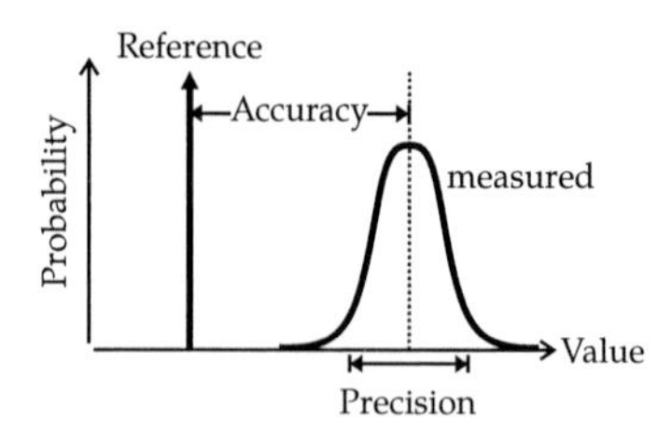

FIGURE 7.7: Precision and accuracy in a measurement.

An imprecise sensing unit is the result of random errors affecting the system functionality. The error spread on the measurements can be due to poor design choices that increase noise effects. Proper circuit design techniques allow to reduce the random errors and therefore increase the precision of a sensor. The accuracy problems are not due to random events but systematic errors, which are those constant or deterministic deviations on the measurement that can be replicated [163] whenever a set of conditions are met.

The non-idealities exhibited by real medical sensing systems caused by process (fixed) and dynamic gain, offset, hysteresis, nonlinearity, cross-sensitivity variations, as well as intrinsic and extrinsic noise sources, deviate the results from the ideal sensor response to the biological parameters or signals of interest. As mentioned earlier in this subsection, the random error components such as noise, causing low precision, are dealt during system design and implementation (i.e., circuit design oriented to noise reduction). Now, in the case of any other predictable error (e.g., temperature gain drift) requires calibration against a reliable reference system (standard) [162]. Dealing with both random and systematic errors ensures that the information gathered from the different sensors in a medical instrument reflects the real physiological quantities under inspection [164].

7.2.3.2 Calibration considerations

Calibration is a critical step required to produce medical devices. Regulators take special care about the requirements for accuracy and precision of a device, and it is normal to find in medical devices standards specifications about the minimum requirements for testing equipment, traceability, and reproducibility [163, 165, 166]. Calibration helps to reduce accuracy issues which, as mentioned earlier, are produced by systematic (predictable) errors. Calibration consists of comparing the sensing unit under study *raw* output with that of a trusted reference system when both are under the same environmental conditions, and equal (controlled) physical quantities applied to their inputs. By performing this comparison over the full measurement input range expected for the sensing unit, as well the environment variations where it has to work typically, it is possible to determine a model for the measuring device accuracy. Therefore, the following aspects have to be taken into account to perform a successful calibration:

- **Accuracy requirements:** Each application has different priorities on the specifications, and this sets the requirements for the calibration procedure. In medical devices, the measurements taken can serve three goals [162]:

- **Diagnosis:** Where the data is continuously compared against a set of value expected ranges. Depending on the range where the measurement falls, a specific diagnosis is determined.
- **Alarm:** The system has to detect if the sensed parameter stays or not within a safe threshold.
- **Titration:** The measurements guide the physicians therapy. The actions over the patient are tuned so that the sensed parameter stays within a target value range.

Each of these goals, together with regulations, impose a required minimum accuracy and precision. Stringent calibration requirements means a complicated and costly process. For instance, the uncertainty of the calibration equipment has to be at least one order of magnitude better than the target accuracy [163], which increases the costs of calibration and hence of the sensing units. Additionally, the number of samples needed per calibration procedure increases (to reduce the effect of random errors) with the target accuracy, leading to larger cycles to obtain the model needed.

- **Mathematical model of the sensing units:** Through literature or experiments, the designer has to model each sensing element in the system mathematically. These models provide insight on the direct sensitivity of the transducers (i.e., the target physiological parameter to measure), dependencies on other physical and environmental parameters (e.g. undesired temperature dependency) as well as cross-sensitivity. Of course, the complexity of these models depends on the target requirements. This information provides an insight into what parameters to control during calibration.
- **Correcting method:** The correction of the systematic errors determined by the calibration procedure are applied as compensation in hardware, software, or in a hybrid manner [164, 167]. Each method has pros and cons; however, in general, hardware compensation methods are more complex and less flexible than the software counterparts.

In the case of IMS, the deployment of the device also has an impact on the accuracy [168]. Detailed understanding of the changes in sensitivity is vital to provide the best solution to achieve the target accuracy and precision.

7.2.3.3 Calibration of pressure sensors

In the case of the present work, the implantable device packaging design eliminates the direct interaction of the electronic components and transducers with the body fluids and tissues (Section 6). Therefore these interactions are not accounted for the calibration of the sensors. However, temperature dependencies, as described earlier in this chapter, play an essential role in the response of the sensor; this is especially relevant for piezoresistive devices. In this way, the calibration goals are to reduce device offset, gain errors (both due to process error in the transducer, interface circuitry and packaging), as well the temperature dependency.

It is important to note that the calibration process has to be done in a post-encapsulation phase since it is expected that the coating layers, applied to protect the device from the harsh body environment, add non-idealities to the sensitivity of the measuring devices. In doing so, the calibration accounts not just for the intrinsic deviations on the transducers and circuitry but on the encapsulation effects on sensitivity and offset.

Off-line Software compensation was chosen as the method to correct the readings' deviations. This selection was based on the software techniques cost-effectiveness, as well as the degree of replication of such methods [167]. Moreover, since the area and power resources in the IMS are limited, it was chosen to apply the correction off-line in the reader hardware. For this, the implant only has to be provided with a small section of nonvolatile memory to store its calibration coefficients (obtained during its calibration procedure). During regular operation, the IMS records and saves to its database *raw* uncompensated data, then when the reader hardware collects the information from the device, it also reads the stored coefficients. Then the compensation can be done using the more powerful computational hardware (and with fewer restrictions on energy usage) on the reader before providing it to the user.

The model for the software compensation had to be defined. Some literature and standards recommend the use of Taylor series [166], however using this method leads to a large number of calibration points [167], making it a complex method for prototyping and proof-of-concept purposes, however, it should not be discarded for a final product device. For the present work, a

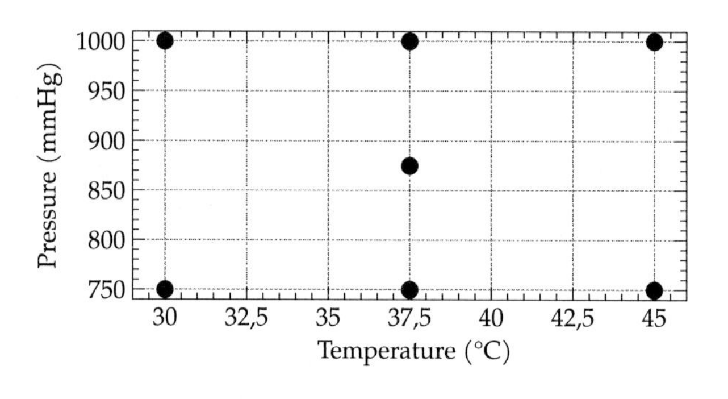

FIGURE 7.8: Selected calibration points (nominal).

rational second-order polynomial approximation [169] was chosen with the form:

$$P(p,t) = a(t)p^2 + b(t)p + c(t) + c_0 \tag{7.1}$$

$$\begin{aligned} a(t) &= a_1t^2 + a_2t \\ b(t) &= b_1t^2 + b_2t \\ c(t) &= c_1t^2 + c_2t \,, \end{aligned} \tag{7.2}$$

where p and t are the uncompensated outputs from the pressure (Section 3) and temperature (Section 4) reading modules, respectively; The functions $a(t)$, $b(t)$ and $c(t)$ are the temperature-dependent coefficients, representing the non-idealities of the transducer, its interface, as well as the effects from the device encapsulation materials.

For the calibration procedure, the setup described in Appendix C was used. The nominal calibration points selected are shown in Figure 7.8. During the procedure, a single implant was placed in the sealed pressure chamber and measurements were taken after about 15 minutes after no change in the chamber's internal temperature was observed, ensuring that all the components are in thermal equilibrium. Each sample taken from the calibration system consisted of the pressure and temperature readings from the reference sensors, and the raw digital output from the pressure and temperature sensors in the IMS (these were read using the `Get single sample` command from Figure 7.6).

Given that the calibration setup can automatically capture the information

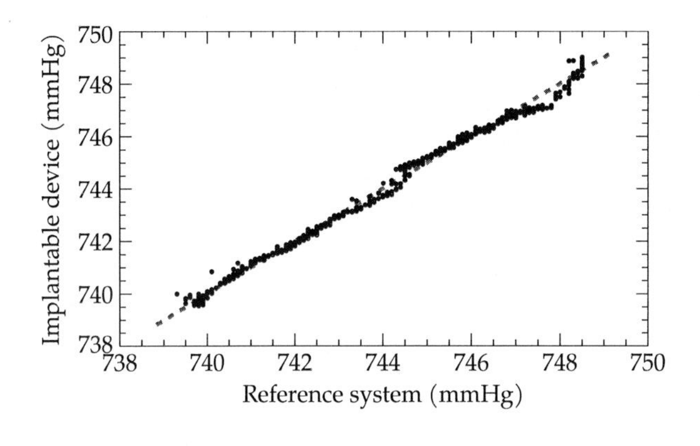

FIGURE 7.9: Calibrated IMS pressure sensor output vs reference system (The dotted line represents the identity curve).

from the reference and IMS sensors, it is possible to record several samples per calibration point. In this way, for each point, 100 samples got recorded and then averaged, reducing variations on the readings (e.g., small changes in the chamber's internal temperature, or leakage). As well, several runs were executed per implant to compare the resulting calibration points. Given that the calibration setup did not include a cooling unit, the procedure starts by fixing the lower temperature and then the pressure is varied, this is repeated for each temperature value. It is relevant to indicate that the final calibration points differed slightly from the ones shown in Figure 7.8 due to external limitations such as an accidentally overheating of the chamber (the setup did not include a cooling system).

Each IMS was calibrated before implantation (and before sterilisation). After a calibration cycle, a long-term test was performed to verify that the system can keep the calibration. Figure 7.9 shows the comparison between a calibrated IMS and a reference system. The curve represents 48 hours of continuous measurement on open-air (atmospheric pressure) and without any controlled temperature, the configured sampling time was 5 minutes. For this specific IMS, the root mean square error (with respect to the reference value) was 0.20 mmHg, which allows for proper measurement of the internal tissue pressure variations (range from -1 mmHg to 60 mmHg as in Section 7.1.1.1).

7.2.4 Reader hardware and software

A reader hardware unit is required to allow physicians and researchers to access the information (and configuration) of an IMS. The interface provided on these devices has to be as simple as possible so that the user gets easy and error-free access to the main functions of the IMS. As well, this interface has to provide transparent information about any exception occurred and warn the user for critical actions.

7.2.4.1 Stand-alone reader unit

A stand-alone reader unit was chosen as the first option for the developed prototype. Figure 7.10 shows a block diagram of this reader unit. As shown, the core of the system was based on a Raspberry Pi module with a light-weight version of Linux. This choice ensures that the user interface could be ported to any other hardware capable of running the operative system Linux. Around the core, a power management unit was implemented to allow the use of a rechargeable lithium-ion battery and a standard micro-USB connector for charging. Also, a real-time clock with an independent battery was used with the idea of keeping the time while the reader hardware was off (the Raspberry Pi module loses the time information when powered off). A 7-inch touchscreen was connected to the core unit to provide the user interface as well for interacting with it. Finally, a break-out board was designed with the required interface circuitry to communicate and charge the IMS.

The Raspberry Pi module was configured as an independent Wi-Fi hotspot so that the user can connect to the reader through this secured network. The SPI and I2C ports were configured as master elements to communicate with the real-time clock and with the touchscreen unit and the IMS interface circuitry, respectively. The host USB was configured to prevent auto-mounting of any USB device.

The user interface was implemented in Python®language. This high-level programming language was chosen due to its high portability and the extensive set of libraries available, as *Tkinter* and *Matplotlib* which were used for the interface front-end. Figure 7.11 shows a screenshot of the reader unit user interface main window, which is only accessed when a valid implantable device is attached to the reader. At start-up, the system provides a simple welcome window with the option to detect an implant, manage files saved or shut down the reader.

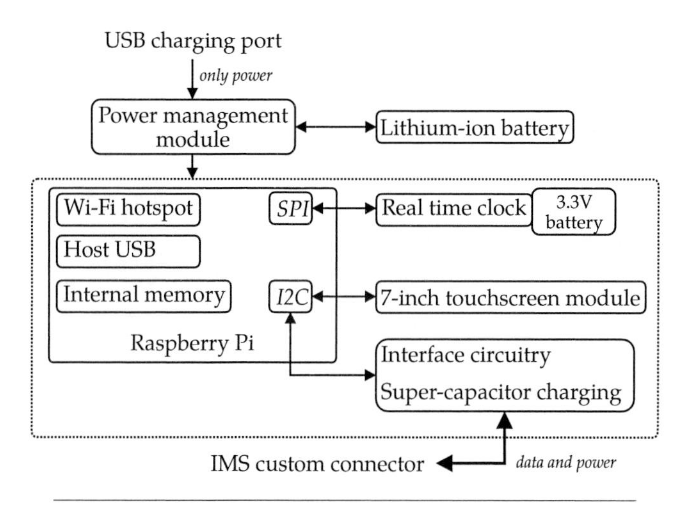

FIGURE 7.10: Block diagram of the reader hardware unit.

The main interface, as shown in Figure 7.11, allows the user to download and preview the data collected from an IMS. For this function, the reader first checks the status of the implant, which carries, among other things, the current measurement cycle, start timestamp, number of samples, and calibration data. In a second step, the full IMS database is collected and verified through a cyclic-redundant code. Once all the information has been retrieved, a temperature compensation algorithm translates the raw data into values of pressure in mmHg and temperature in °C. The output of this compensation function is stored together with the IMS ID, timestamp, and other status information into a comma-separated file. Besides, the compensated data is used for the user interface preview pane.

The user also has the option to adjust the reader hardware date and time (used to calculate the IMS timestamp) and to change the sampling time of the implant (configuration option). A control for *live mode* is accessible from the main window. This mode can be used to debug the IMS, as well as to check its functionality immediately after a successful implantation procedure.

The *Start new measurement* option is used to set ready the IMS for a new measurement cycle. By clicking this last option, the reader hardware sets as new IMS timestamp the current date and time. Besides, as part of the actions taken, a `Clear database` command is sent to the implantable unit to clear the content of the data memory and its status registers. This action as well closes

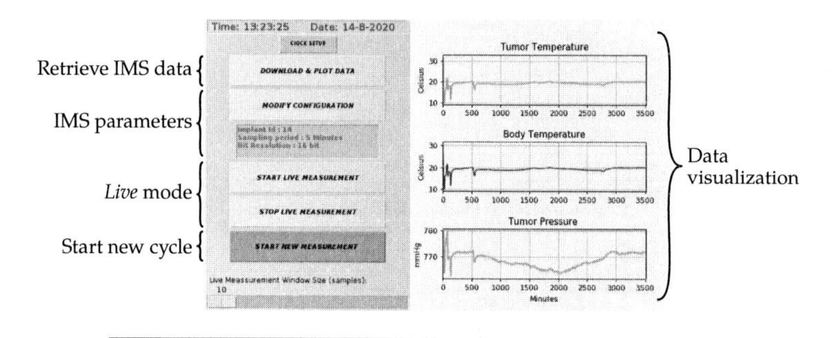

FIGURE 7.11: User interface main window in the IMS reader hardware unit.

the main interface until a new IMS is connected.

Data security

With the proliferation of IMS, security concerns are a hot topic nowadays. However, due to the tight requirements on size and energy consumption, the use of standard cryptographic methods is not always possible, and several custom solutions have to be used. The concerns about IMS data security depend on the type of implantable system. In the case of units that actuate over the body (e.g., electrical stimulator devices and drug deliver units, among others), the main threat is that a malicious attack to the IMS can result in the application of a lethal dose to the patient.

Regarding monitoring IMS (as in the present work), data security should allow to preserve the fundamental human right of protection and privacy of personal, genomic, and health information. The convenience of having a device that can continuously monitor health and response to treatment has opened a new paradigm for information security: the patient carries the information that typically was physically restricted to a laboratory or hospital. This advantage could also be a weakness for IMS since unauthorised individuals can potentially access this data. Because of this, information security measures have to be implemented in the communication link and the storage units involved.

As previously described, the developed prototype makes use of a wired link to communicate with the reader unit (Section 7.2.2). The security risks on wired connections are reduced when compared to their wireless counterparts.

In this way, critical commands as `Set configuration` were protected by a second verification word. This parameter is passed to the device by the reader hardware the first time the system is used and therefore links the implant to a specific reader interface.

In the developed reader interface, the data captured from the implantable device is stored on its internal memory. Two security measures were taken to protect this information from unauthorised access. First, the user has to log into the private Wi-Fi network of the reader unit (with a hidden SSID), which is password protected. Second, once the user is logged into the private network, it has to access a secure web page provided hosted in the reader hardware. This web page requires a second password to access it. After the user has passed these two filters, they can copy the files stored in the reader unit.

Once the information is retrieved into the user's computer (usually the physician or researcher), the security of it depends on the internal protocols followed by the health or research facility where the experiments are done. However, this is not a critical point for the work presented here, since the purpose of these prototypes is to prove the concept of this implantable device and complementary units. Nevertheless, for future developments the security of this information has to be checked from all the mentioned angles: IMS, communication link, reader hardware, as well any device where this information has to be stored.

7.2.5 Proof-of-concept results

For the proof-of-concept, an in-vivo test was performed in cooperation with the Institut für Anatomie und Experimentelle Morphologie from the Universitätsklinikum Hamburg-Eppendorf (UKE). The laboratories from UKE have access to mice with Severe Combined Immunodeficiency (SCID) and several cancer-cell lines that are used in their research tasks. An animal ethics committee approved the experiments described in Hamburg on January 30th 2019.

The research team from UKE prepared four experiments with PC3 xenograft models on SCID-mice (prostate cancer cell line). However, due to problems related to the SCID-mice (generation of skin ulcers), several tests had to be cancelled before implantation. The previous problem happened as well in both successful implantations, two days after each procedure. As per the

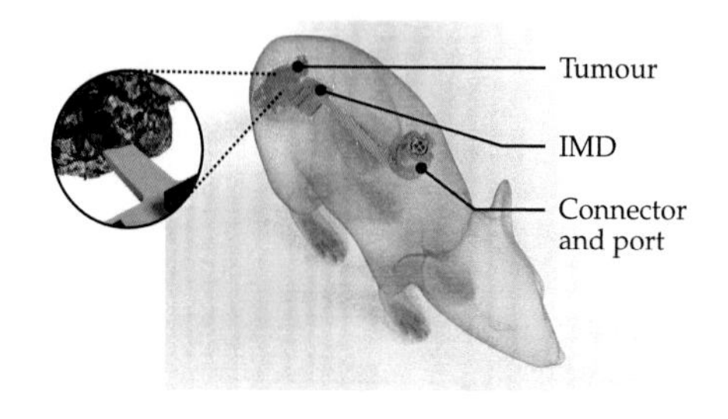

FIGURE 7.12: Graphical representation of the IMS during in vivo test.

ethical responsibility agreed, the experiments had to be stopped if skin ulcers, reduced mobility or a tumour size larger than 1.5 cm, were observed.

In the case of the two successful experiments, the cancerous tumour models were left to grow for about two weeks until reaching a size of 1 cm. At this point, the UKE researchers proceeded with the implantation procedure as planned (Section 6.3). Figure 7.12 shows a graphical representation (we agreed to avoid pictures of the real animals) of the tumour and IMS locations in the mouse. The implant port was located on the upper back of the animal. After the implantation procedure, and while the mouse was still sedated, the reader hardware unit was used to verify the IMS functionality and in addition to charging the device for its first measurement cycle.

During the experiments, a barometer with a resolution of 0.05 mmHg was placed in the cage with the mouse. The readings from this barometer (accompanied by a timestamp) were used later in post-processing to remove the variations on atmospheric pressure from the values recorded by the IMS.

The implanted systems were able to run autonomously for more than 48 hours at a sampling rate of 5 minutes. Figure 7.13 and 7.14 present the results for pressure and temperature obtained from the two successful runs. The presented results are not filtered and also show noise and artefacts from the animal movement. An *approximation* curve was also plotted together with the gathered data. This tendency curve is the result of a denoise wavelet algorithm applied in Matlab®.

Figure 7.13 corresponds to the relative pressure measurement obtained from the in vivo tests (i.e., the difference between pressure data from the IMS and the external barometer). As shown in the figure, the data presents large

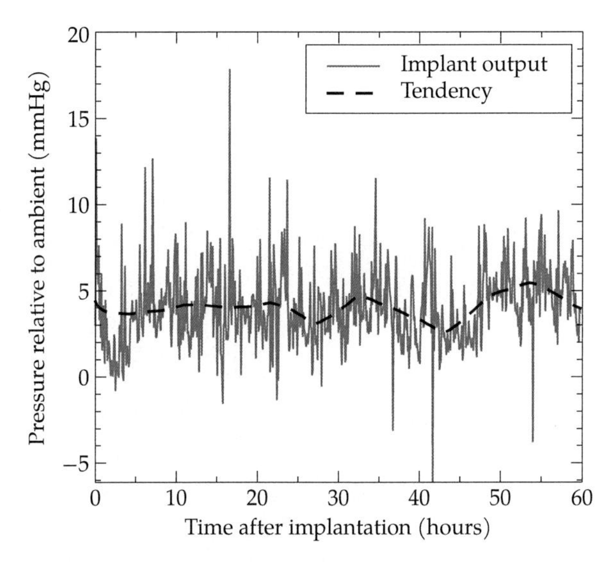

(a) First experiment round - PC3 cell line (February 6th 2019).

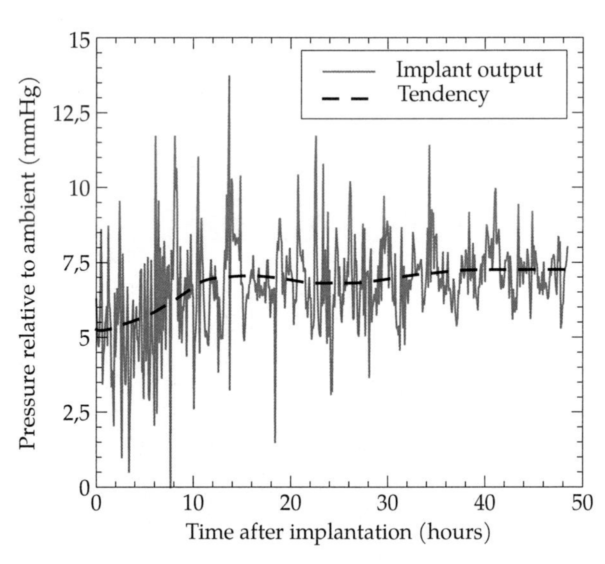

(b) Second experiment round - PC3 cell line (November 4th 2019).

FIGURE 7.13: Pressure readings captured during in-vivo experiments.

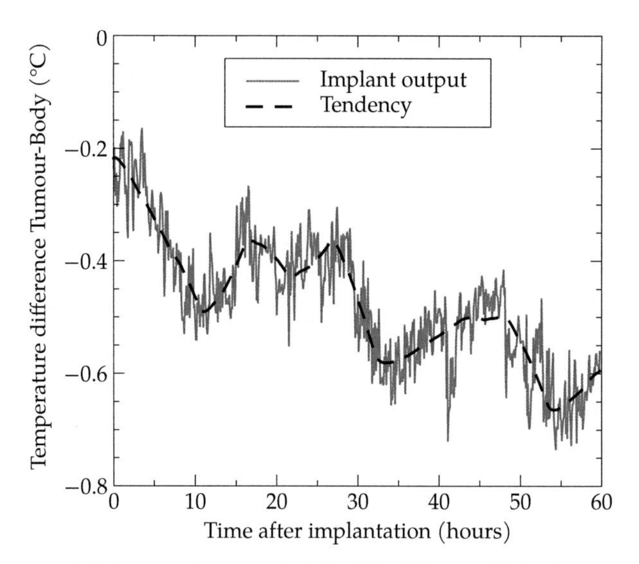

(a) First experiment round - PC3 cell line (February 6th 2019).

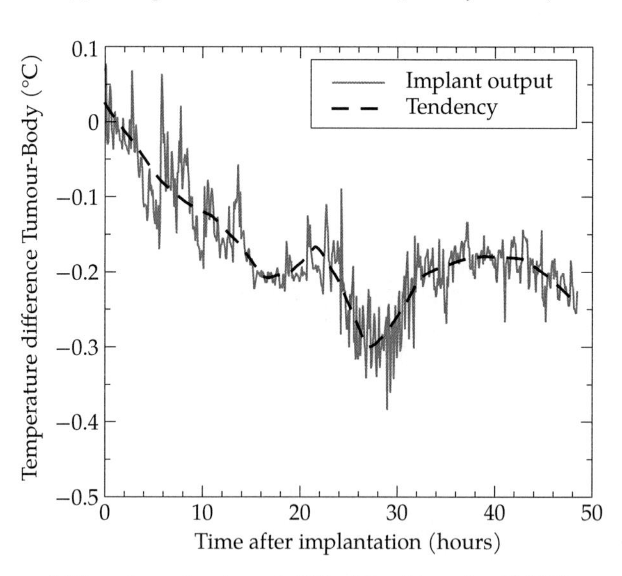

(b) Second experiment round - PC3 cell line (November 4th 2019).

FIGURE 7.14: Temperature readings captured during in-vivo experiments.

spikes which are mainly the result of artefacts due to the animal movement. These spikes are a problem caused by the use of a single absolute pressure transducer in the IMS. However, by applying the wavelet denoise algorithm, it is possible to extract the low-frequency components from the data to generate a tendency curve. Relevant from these curves is that over time there is an appreciable increase of the tumour pressure, which, as per the theory relative to the cancer microenvironment Section 7.1.2, is evidence of a developing tumour.

The dataset presented in Figure 7.13.b shows the recorded difference of temperature between the inside and outside of the tumour. As shown in the figure, both datasets present, over time, a decrease in the tumour temperature relative to its body temperature. These results are consistent with those from a growing tumour in [157, 159] (briefly described in Section 7.1.3).

The two experiments described were executed without the application of any therapy on the mice, meaning that it was expected for the tumour to have continuous growth and development. As pointed out, in both experiments, the temperature and pressure readings showed the expected behaviour for a growing tumour, which serves as the first proof-of-concept.

Chapter 8

Conclusion and Outlook

This work presented the foundations for autonomous data acquisition on an implantable medical system for the measurement of pressure and temperature in tumours. Considerations for obtaining biophysical parameters were analysed and tested by the implementation of mixed-signal interfaces on ASIC. The trade-offs between performance and noise, silicon area usage, and energy consumption, for interfaces in implantable systems, were discussed and experimentally verified.

Three ASIC were fabricated to verify the time keeping, data acquisition interfaces and on-chip temperature sensor developed during this work. Two interfaces were implemented for the pressure sensing in IMS to demonstrate the potential and trade-offs of both capacitive and piezoresistive pressure transducers. The interface for capacitive pressure transducers was implemented in 350 nm CMOS technology occupying an area of 0.055 mm^2. With this interface, a maximum resolution of 0.3 mmHg (using a commercially available transducer) was achieved while consuming a maximum of 20 µW during conversion (full range conversion). Furthermore, a study was presented on the development of an interface for piezoresistive pressure sensors. The design criteria for the conversion path were presented. As an initial step to develop an interface for this type of sensors, a sigma-delta modulator was implemented in 180 nm CMOS technology, occupying an area of 0.058 mm^2. The developed modulator presented an ENOB of 9.4070 bits (SNR of 58.39 dB) for a bandwidth of 1.953 kHz (OSR of 512). The measured power consumption of the modulator, during operation, was 167.32 µW.

The on-chip temperature transducer implemented in 180 nm CMOS technology reached an average sensitivity of $-4.7463\,\mathrm{mV\,{}^{\circ}C^{-1}}$. Process variations resulted in an average deviation of 117.56 ppm on the measured sensitivity in the test chips. Finally, the power and area utilisation for this transducer are 927 nW (during operation) and 0.012 mm^2, respectively.

In addition to the sensing units, a low-power and low frequency timing unit was developed. This unit provides a base sampling time of 34.45 s with a variation of around 0.63 s. This sampling period is realised with a power consumption of 1.98 nW. Additionally, the developed unit provides a clock gating and generation unit.

An implantable medical system prototype was implemented for in-vivo tests. The designed implantable system can acquire periodic samples of pressure and temperature from a tumour. The use of a low-power timer to keep track of the sampling enabled the system to run autonomously for more than 48 hours from the energy stored in a super-capacitor bank.

A combination of medical-grade silicone and parylene-c was used to encapsulate the implantable system. This encapsulation successfully protected from each other the electronics and the host animal during the in-vivo experiments. The encapsulation application, the miniature connector fabrication, and even the design of the implant geometry benefited from additive manufacturing techniques.

The in vivo-tests verified the concept for the implantable system under research and development. The pressure and temperature measured from the cancer xenografts were consistent with the expected values for a growing tumour. These results provide confidence to continue development of this implant, furnishing physicians and researchers fighting cancer with an effective tool.

8.1 Future work

The implantable system prototype system was successful in continuously recording the temperature and pressure from the cancer xenografts in the in-vivo experiments. However, the presented work represents only the first steps towards an implantable system for clinical use, and several enhancements to the presented prototype will be necessary. The recommendations for the future design steps for this system are summarised here:

As discussed in Section 3.2.2, the proposed interface for capacitive transducers presents various improvement opportunities. In the case of the TDC, its design was over-dimensioned to decrease its influence on the novel CTC characterisation. Therefore, based on the CTC results and the target resolution, both the oscillator and digital counter can be optimised. Additionally, to further reduce the power consumption, a dual supply voltage scheme can be implemented in the CDC. While the supply voltage in the CTC can be kept between 3.3 V to 2.7 V, the blocks in the TDC can be powered from a much lower supply rail. Such a configuration would save dynamic power; however, care has to be taken in order to reduce the effect on the jitter introduced by the oscillator.

Section 3.2.1 presented a simple interface for piezoresistive pressure sensors. This concept represents our first steps towards a high-resolution low-power interface for piezoresistive transducers based on a sigma-delta ADC that replaces the previous test interface. A low-noise low-power analogue front-end should be implemented to complete this interface. The designed AFE has to provide offset compensation, as well as the option to adjust its gain. Regarding the Sigma-Delta ADC, a decimator and digital filter are required to complete the interface. Furthermore, improvements on the layout routing of the modulator, as well as the use of a fully differential OTA could elicit better performance from this block.

The prototype presented in this work used a wired link for data and power transmission. However, this kind of connection, though robust, reduces the comfort of the individual wearing it, and it is not an option for a commercial device for human use. Hence, this interface must be replaced by a secure wireless link. The link ought to offer enough power to charge the supercapacitor bank in a reasonable time as well. Finally, such a link will need to provide a high level of security to keep the patient's sensitive information safe.

Full integration of the processing, energy management and communication blocks shown in Figure 2.1 is required for achieving the goal of a miniaturised system capable of being implanted via a biopsy needle. Furthermore, smaller but dense energy storage elements, such as thin solid-state batteries must be explored.

Appendix A

Low Power PVT-Independent Current Source

Current references are critical blocks in the design of analogue circuits. These construction blocks have to present stable value independent of temperature, supply, and fabrication process variations. The most common implementation to obtain such a stable current reference is to use a band-gap reference (BGR) circuit [59]. However, these circuits are not suitable for the nano ampere-range currents required in low-power biomedical devices. This section presents a low-power current reference circuit able to provide reference values in the

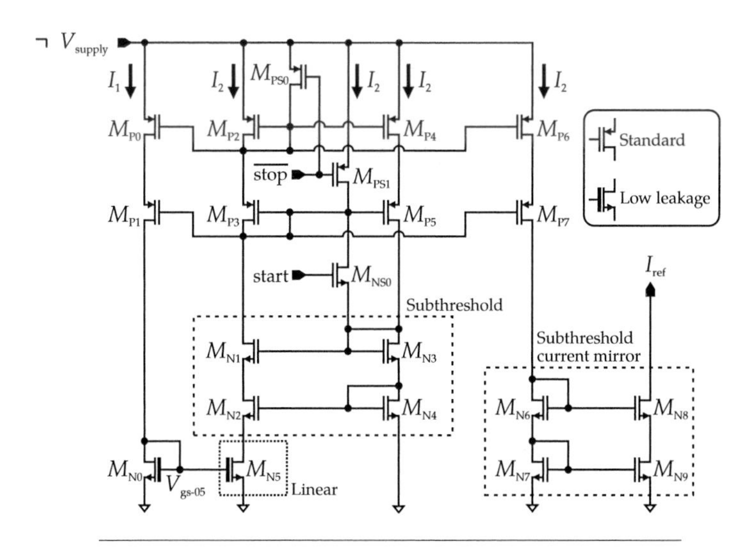

FIGURE A.1: Schematic view of the implemented current reference.

nano ampere range. The sensing interfaces developed in this work make use of the unit presented in this section.

Figure A.1 shows the schematic view of the current reference developed during this work. The system makes only use of CMOS devices. Except for transistors M_{N0} and M_{N5}, which are low leakage NMOS transistors, all the transistors used are from the standard process (i.e. AMS 350 nm). This design is an improvement from Oguey's design [170]. In the proposed system, transistors M_{N1}, M_{N2}, M_{N3}, M_{N4}, as well those used in the current mirror, are biased in subthreshold mode. Furthermore, the low-leakage transistor M_{N5} is biased in the linear region, with a drain-source voltage dependent on the difference between the gate voltage on transistors M_{N2} and M_{N4} (both in subthreshold region):

$$\begin{aligned} V_{\text{ds-MN5}} &= V_{\text{gs-MN4}} - V_{\text{gs-MN2}} \\ &= nV_T \ln\left(\frac{W_{\text{MN2}} L_{\text{MN4}}}{L_{\text{MN2}} W_{\text{MN4}}}\right) + \left(V_{\text{th-MN4}} - V_{\text{th-MN2}}\right) . \end{aligned} \tag{A.1}$$

Additionally, the drain current of transistors M_{N0} (diode connected) and M_{N5} (linear region) define the currents I_1 and I_2, respectively, by the following relationships:

$$I_1 = I_{\text{d-MN0}} = \frac{\mu C_{ox}}{2} \frac{W_{\text{MN0}}}{L_{\text{MN0}}} (V_{\text{gs-MN0}} - V_{\text{th-MN0}})^2 \tag{A.2}$$

$$I_2 = I_{\text{d-MN5}} = \mu C_{ox} \frac{W_{\text{MN5}}}{L_{\text{MN5}}} (V_{\text{gs-MN5}} - V_{\text{th-MN5}}) V_{\text{ds-MN5}} . \tag{A.3}$$

By making the ration W/L equal on both M_{N0} and M_{N5}, currents I1 and I2 can be related to each other by:

$$I_1 = \alpha I_2 , \tag{A.4}$$

with the proportionality constant α calculated as:

$$\alpha = \frac{V_{\text{gs-05}} - V_{\text{th-ll}}}{2V_{\text{ds-MN5}}} , \tag{A.5}$$

where $V_{\text{th-ll}}$ is the threshold voltage for the NMOS low leakage transistors M_{N0} and M_{N5}, and $V_{\text{gs-05}}$ is the gate voltage for both transistors.

Furthermore, a relation between the drain-to-source voltage of M_{N5} and $V_{\text{gs-05}} - V_{\text{th-ll}}$ is obtained by differentiating with respect to the temperature

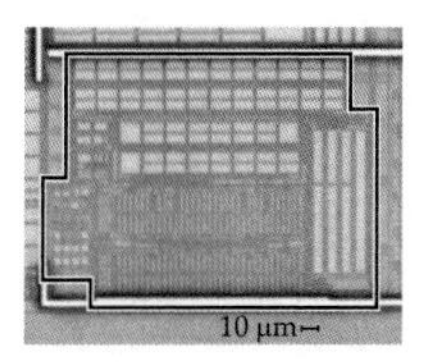

FIGURE A.2: Annotated micrograph of the implemented current reference circuit.

the natural logarithm of expressions Equations A.2 and A.3:

$$\frac{1}{V_{\text{ds-MN5}}}\frac{\delta V_{\text{ds-MN5}}}{\delta T} = \frac{1}{V_{\text{gs-05}} - V_{\text{th-ll}}}\frac{\delta(V_{\text{gs-05}} - V_{\text{th-ll}})}{\delta T} . \quad \text{(A.6)}$$

In this way, it is possible to define a value for α (Equation A.5) and the W/L ratios for transistors M_{N2} and M_{N4} (Equation A.1) that satisfy the previous expression to design a PVT-independent current source.

This current reference was implemented in AMS 350 nm CMOS technology, as part of the test ASIC presented in Appendix B.1. Figure A.2 shows an annotated micrograph of this implementation. The design shown corresponds to the current reference used for the CDC presented in Section 3.2.2.2. The target value for the reference current was 1 nA. Experimental results showed that the current reference value was 1.144 nA in average. Table A.1 presents a summary of the results from the implemented current reference circuit. Further detail on these results were presented in the publication [171].

TABLE A.1: Summary results for the implemented current reference unit.

Parameter	Measured
Supply (**V**)	2.7 - 3.3
Iref (**nA**)	1.144
Power (μ**W**)	2.1 2.7 V
Temperature coefficient* (**ppm**/°**C**)	485
Line regulation (%/**V**)	0.11
Load regulation (%/**V**)	0.81
Area (**mm**^{2})	0.02

* Values measured in the range 27 °C to 44 °C.

Appendix B

Fabricated ASICs

B.1 TEST ASIC I

- **Technology:** AMS 350nm CMOS
- **Fabrication date:** Oct. 2017
- **Dimensions:** 2332x1948 μm^2

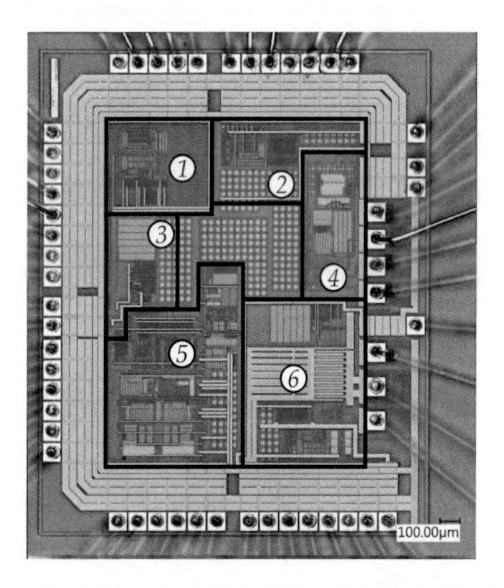

FIGURE B.1: Annotated micrograph of the test ASIC II. 1. Capacitance to digital converter, 2. Timer and clock generation unit, 3. Low power LDO, 4. Wireless power harvesting unit. 5. Piezoresistive sensor interface (AFE+ADC), 6. Data transmission unit.

B.2 TEST ASIC II

- **Technology:** X-FAB 180nm CMOS
- **Fabrication date:** May. 2019
- **Dimensions:** 2332x1948 μm^2

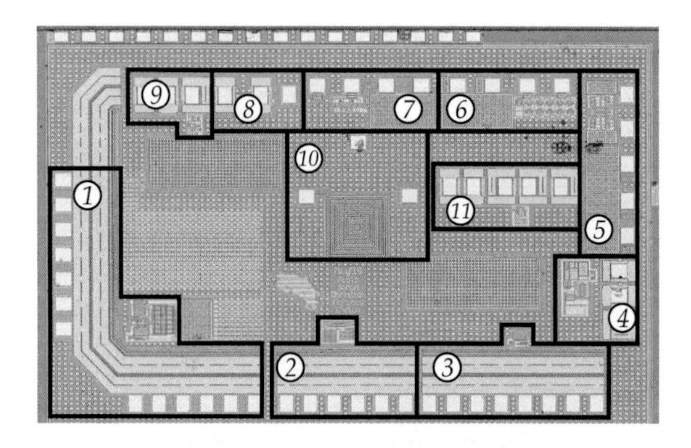

FIGURE B.2: Annotated micrograph of the test ASIC III. 1. Sigma delta modulator, 2. Temperature sensor, 3. OTA for sigma delta modulator, 4. LDO *high power*, 5. AC/DC converter v1.2, 6. AC/DC converter v2, 7. AC/DC converter v1, 8. Low-power voltage reference, 9. LDO *low power*, 10. On-Chip coil, 11. Low power amplifier.

B.3 TEST ASIC III

- **Technology:** X-FAB 180nm CMOS
- **Fabrication date:** Jan. 2020
- **Dimensions:** 3120x3120 μm^2

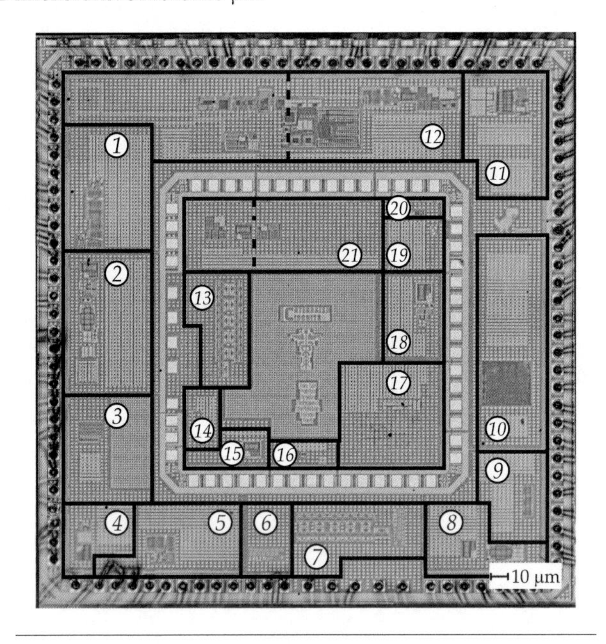

FIGURE B.3: Annotated micrograph of the test ASIC III. 1. Sigma delta modulator, 2. Temperature sensor, 3. OTA for sigma delta modulator, 4. LDO *high power*, 5. AC/DC converter v1.2, 6. AC/DC converter v2, 7. AC/DC converter v1, 8. Low-power voltage reference, 9. LDO *low power*, 10. On-Chip coil, 11. Low power amplifier.

Appendix C

Test system with variable pressure and temperature

A test and calibration setup was required for the development of the system. First of all, there was need of a chamber that could withstand a pressure of more than 1000mmHg. Also, a way to generate and accurately measure the pressure was required. Furthermore, the system had to be able to set an internal temperature for the tests. This last point was relevant for the setup for two reasons: The IMD had also to measure temperature, and second, the pressure sensors (transducer and interfaces) have temperature dependencies that required characterisation.

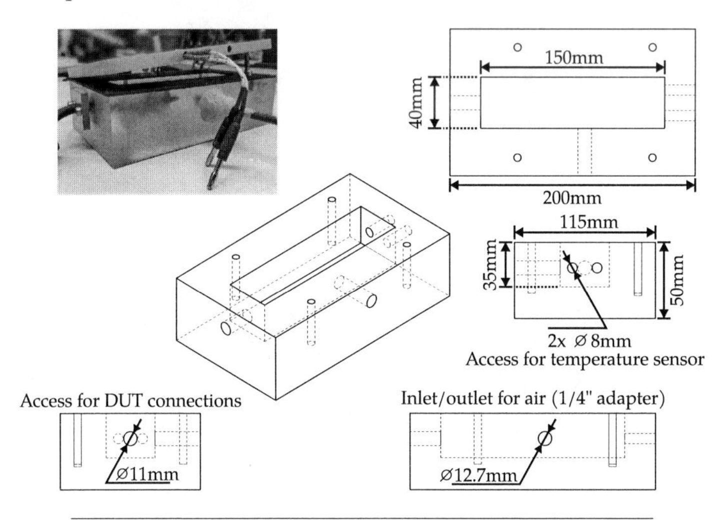

FIGURE C.1: Pressure chamber diagram and picture.

The core of the setup was based on the pressure chamber shown in Figure C.1. The chamber was fabricated in acrylic glass (using CNC milling). The chamber also had a metal lid (as shown in the picture) with heating elements attached to it. The lid attaches to the chamber by four screws. A ring of rubber in between the chamber body and the lid works as a hermetic seal. The chamber body has two holes in one side to provide access to pt100 temperature probes. Furthermore, a third opening allows to get access to connections to the device under test (DUT). Furthermore, there is a slot to use a standard 1/2" adapter for the application of pressure or vacuum.

Two variants of the test setup were used. The first option used a Mensor CPA2501 calibrator together with a manual pump. This setup is shown in Figure C.2.a. The second setup, shown in fig Figure C.2.b instead used a Fluke-719Pro30G (which includes a digitally controlled pump). Both setups used a Raspberry pi to capture the sensor data and the reference systems data (Mensor CPA2501 or Fluke-719Pro30G). A wireless remote server was configured in the raspberry pin to display and control the system from a PC (as visible in the figures). The outputs from each test were saved in CSV files for post-processing.

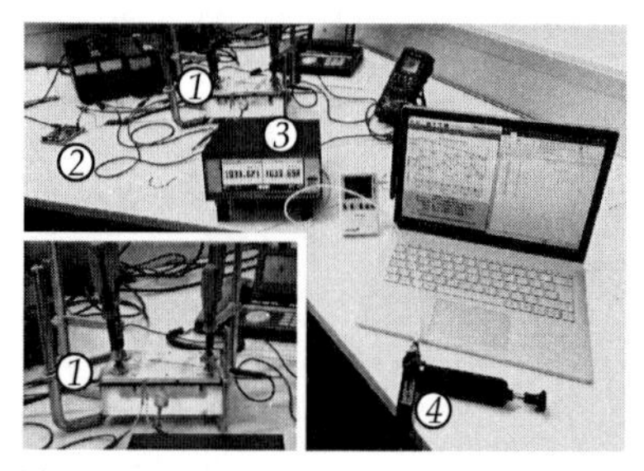

(a) Using Mensor CPA2501 pressure calibrator.

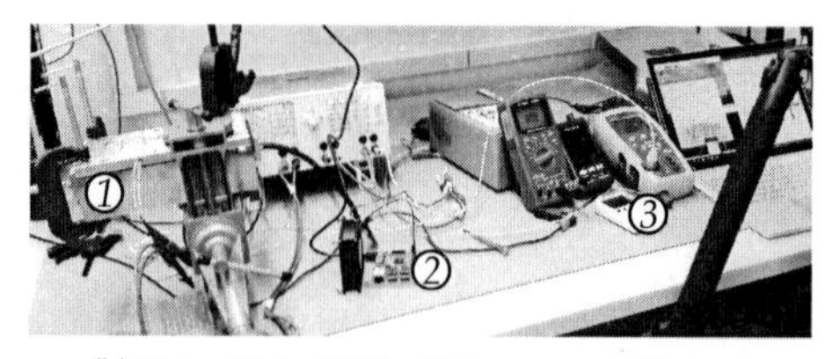

(b) Using Fluke-719Pro30G pressure calibrator.

FIGURE C.2: Annotated picture of the test setups for pressure and temperature tests. 1. Pressure chamber, 2. Raspberry-pi (data acquisition), 3. Pressure calibrator, 4. Manual pump.

Bibliography

[1] *WHO report on cancer: setting priorities, investing wisely and providing care for all*. 2020.

[2] M. A. Hayat. *Methods of Cancer Diagnosis, Therapy and Prognosis*. Vol. Volume 2: General Methods and Overviews, Lung Carcinoma and Prostate Carcinoma. Dordrecht: Springer Netherlands, 2008. ISBN: 978-1-4020-8441-6. DOI: 10.1007/978-1-4020-8442-3.

[3] European Health Information Gateway. *Computed Tomography Scanners (equipments per 100000 population)*. URL: https://gateway.euro.who.int/en/indicators/hlthres_37-computed-tomography-scanners-per-100-000/ (visited on 14/07/2020).

[4] European Health Information Gateway. *Magnetic Resonance Imaging Units (equipments per 100000 population)*. URL: https://gateway.euro.who.int/en/indicators/hlthres_95-magnetic-resonance-imaging-units-per-100-000/ (visited on 14/07/2020).

[5] *Diagnostics: Blood pressure, 1881*. URL: https://wellcomecollection.org/works/zg7yefyu (visited on 27/04/2020). Attribution 4.0 International (CC BY 4.0).

[6] Joseph F. Dyro. *Clinical engineering handbook*. Academic Press series in biomedical engineering. Amsterdam: Elsevier/Acad. Press, 2004. ISBN: 9780122265709. URL: http://site.ebrary.com/lib/alltitles/docDetail.action?docID=10128020.

[7] Vinod Kumar Khanna. *Implantable Medical Electronics*. Cham: Springer International Publishing, 2016. ISBN: 978-3-319-25446-3. DOI: 10.1007/978-3-319-25448-7.

[8] Mark N. Gasson, Eleni Kosta and Diana M. Bowman. *Human ICT implants: Technical, legal and ethical considerations*. Vol. 23. Information Technology and Law Series. The Hague: T. M. C. Asser Press, 2012. ISBN: 9789067048699. DOI: 10.1007/978-90-6704-870-5. URL: http://site.ebrary.com/lib/alltitles/docDetail.action?docID=10574406.

[9] P. Gerrish et al. 'Challenges and constraints in designing implantable medical ICs'. In: *IEEE Transactions on Device and Materials Reliability* 5.3 (2005), pp. 435–444. ISSN: 1558-2574. DOI: 10.1109/TDMR.2005.858914.

[10] Arthur H.M. van Roermund, Herman Casier and Michiel Steyaert. *Analog Circuit Design*. Dordrecht: Springer Netherlands, 2006. ISBN: 978-1-4020-5185-2. DOI: 10.1007/1-4020-5186-7.

[11] Scott Makeig et al. *Towards a New Cognitive Neuroscience: Modeling Natural Brain Dynamics*. s.l.: Frontiers Media SA, 2014. ISBN: 9782889192717. URL: http://www.doabooks.org/doab?func=fulltext&rid=17779.

[12] Lawrence Yu, Brian J. Kim and Ellis Meng. 'Chronically implanted pressure sensors: challenges and state of the field'. In: *Sensors (Basel, Switzerland)* 14.11 (2014), pp. 20620–20644. DOI: 10.3390/s141120620.

[13] Elias Greenbaum and David Zhou. *Implantable Neural Prostheses 1*. New York, NY: Springer US, 2009. ISBN: 978-0-387-77260-8. DOI: 10.1007/978-0-387-77261-5.

[14] Elena P. Ivanova, Kateryna Bazaka and Russell J. Crawford. *New functional biomaterials for medicine and healthcare*. Vol. 67. Woodhead Publishing series in biomaterials. Oxford et al.: Woodhead Publishing, 2014. ISBN: 9781782422655.

[15] David A. Rubenstein, Wei Yin and Mary D. Frame. *Biofluid mechanics: An introduction to fluid mechanics, macrocirculation, and microcirculation*. Academic Press series in biomedical engineering. Amsterdam: Elsevier, 2012. ISBN: 9780123813831. DOI: 10.1016/C2009-0-61089-8.

[16] Carl-Henrik Heldin et al. 'High interstitial fluid pressure - an obstacle in cancer therapy'. In: *Nature reviews. Cancer* 4.10 (2004), pp. 806–813. ISSN: 1474-175X. DOI: 10.1038/nrc1456.

[17] Gianfranco Baronzio et al. 'Tumor interstitial fluid as modulator of cancer inflammation, thrombosis, immunity and angiogenesis'. In: *Anticancer research* 32.2 (2012), pp. 405–414.

[18] Gianfranco Baronzio, Christopher R. Cogle and Gianfranco Fiorentini. *Cancer Microenvironment and Therapeutic Implications: Tumor Pathophysiology Mechanisms and Therapeutic Strategies*. 1st ed. Dordrecht: Springer Netherlands, 2009. ISBN: 978-1-4020-9575-7. DOI: 10.1007/978-1-4020-9576-4.

[19] L. J. Liu et al. 'Phenomenological model of interstitial fluid pressure in a solid tumor'. In: *Physical review. E, Statistical, nonlinear, and soft matter physics* 84.2 Pt 1 (2011), p. 021919. DOI: 10.1103/PhysRevE.84.021919.

[20] Robert W. Schrier. *Manual of nephrology*. 7. Aufl. Philadelphia: Lippincott Williams & Wilkins, 2009. ISBN: 9780781796194. URL: http://ovidsp.ovid.com/ovidweb.cgi?T=JS&NEWS=n&CSC=Y&PAGE=booktext&D=books&AN=01435375.

[21] Kenneth D. McClatchey. *Clinical laboratory medicine*. 2nd ed. Philadelphia: Lippincott Wiliams & Wilkins, 2002. ISBN: 0683307517. URL: http://ovidsp.ovid.com/ovidweb.cgi?T=JS&PAGE=booktext&NEWS=N&DF=bookdb&AN=00149848/2nd_Edition/3&XPATH=/PG(0).

[22] M. M. Thompson and Robert Fitridge, eds. *Mechanisms of vascular disease: A reference book for vascular specialists*. [Updated ed.] Adelaide: Barr Smith Press, 2011. ISBN: 9780987171825. DOI: 10.20851/j.ctt1sq5w94.

[23] *Engraving: direct sphymograph; E.J. Marey*. URL: https://wellcomecollection.org/works/qsfjbt8m (visited on 27/04/2020). Attribution 4.0 International (CC BY 4.0).

[24] J. Booth. 'A short history of blood pressure measurement'. In: *Proceedings of the Royal Society of Medicine* 70.11 (1977), pp. 793–799. ISSN: 0035-9157.

[25] Stephen Hales et al. *Haemastatics*. London: Printed for W. Innys and R. Manby, at the west-end of St. Paul's, and T. Woodward, at the Half-Moon between Temple-Gate, Fleetstreet, 1733. DOI: 10.5962/bhl.title.106596.

[26] Rüdiger Kramme, Klaus-Peter Hoffmann and Robert S. Pozos. *Springer handbook of medical technology*. Berlin: Springer, 2011. ISBN: 978-3-540-74657-7. DOI: 10.1007/978-3-540-74658-4.

[27] Florian Rader and Ronald G. Victor. 'The Slow Evolution of Blood Pressure Monitoring: But Wait, Not So Fast!' In: *JACC: Basic to Translational Science* 2.6 (2017), pp. 643–645. DOI: 10.1016/j.jacbts.2017.11.001.

[28] *IEEE Standard for a Smart Transducer Interface for Sensors and Actuators - Digital Communication and Transducer Electronic Data Sheet (TEDS) Formats for Distributed Multidrop Systems*. Piscataway, NJ, USA, 2003. DOI: 10.1109/IEEESTD.2004.94443.

[29] Marc J. Madou. *Fundamentals of Microfabrication: The Science of Miniaturization, Second Edition*. 2nd ed. London: Chapman and Hall/CRC, 2002. ISBN: 9780849308260.

[30] Stephen A. Dyer. *Wiley Survey of Instrumentation and Measurement*. Hoboken: John Wiley & Sons Inc, 2004. ISBN: 9780471394846.

[31] Charles S. Smith. 'Piezoresistance Effect in Germanium and Silicon'. In: *Physical Review* 94.1 (1954), pp. 42–49. ISSN: 0031-899X. DOI: 10.1103/PhysRev.94.42.

[32] O. N. Tufte, P. W. Chapman and Donald Long. 'Silicon Diffused-Element Piezoresistive Diaphragms'. In: *Journal of Applied Physics* 33.11 (1962), pp. 3322–3327. ISSN: 0021-8979. DOI: 10.1063/1.1931164.

[33] A. Gieles. 'Subminiature silicon pressure transducer'. In: *1969 IEEE International Solid-State Circuits Conference. Digest of Technical Papers*. IEEE, 2/19/1969 - 2/21/1969, pp. 108–109. DOI: 10.1109/ISSCC.1969.1154778.

[34] S. Santosh Kumar and B. D. Pant. 'Design principles and considerations for the 'ideal' silicon piezoresistive pressure sensor: a focused review'. In: *Microsystem Technologies* 20.7 (2014), pp. 1213–1247. ISSN: 0946-7076. DOI: 10.1007/s00542-014-2215-7.

[35] A. Alvin Barlian et al. 'Review: Semiconductor Piezoresistance for Microsystems'. In: *Proceedings of the IEEE. Institute of Electrical and Electronics Engineers* 97.3 (2009), pp. 513–552. ISSN: 0018-9219. DOI: 10.1109/JPROC.2009.2013612.

[36] Jan G. Korvink and Oliver Paul. *MEMS: A Practical Guide to Design, Analysis, and Applications*. Berlin, Heidelberg: Springer Berlin Heidelberg, 2006. ISBN: 978-3-540-21117-4. DOI: 10.1007/978-3-540-33655-6.

[37] S. Santosh Kumar and B. D. Pant. 'Erratum to: Design principles and considerations for the 'ideal' silicon piezoresistive pressure sensor: a focused review'. In: *Microsystem Technologies* 20.12 (2014), p. 2303. ISSN: 0946-7076. DOI: 10.1007/s00542-014-2289-2.

[38] Winncy Y. Du. *Resistive, Capacitive, Inductive, and Magnetic Sensor Technologies*. CRC Press, 2014. ISBN: 9780429093180. DOI: 10.1201/b17685.

[39] M. Habibi et al. 'A surface micromachined capacitive absolute pressure sensor array on a glass substrate'. In: *Sensors and Actuators A: Physical* 46.1-3 (1995), pp. 125–128. ISSN: 09244247. DOI: 10.1016/0924-4247(94)00874-H.

[40] D. Brox, A. R. Mohammadi and K. Takahata. 'Non-lithographically microfabricated capacitive pressure sensor for biomedical applications'. In: *Electronics Letters* 47.18 (2011), p. 1015. ISSN: 00135194. DOI: 10.1049/el.2011.2230.

[41] Y. Zhang et al. 'A high-sensitive ultra-thin MEMS capacitive pressure sensor'. In: *2011 16th International Solid-State Sensors, Actuators and Microsystems Conference*. IEEE, 5.06.2011 - 09.06.2011, pp. 112–115. ISBN: 978-1-4577-0157-3. DOI: 10.1109/TRANSDUCERS.2011.5969151.

[42] Madhurima Chattopadhyay and Debjyoti Chowdhury. 'Design and performance analysis of MEMS capacitive pressure sensor array for measurement of heart rate'. In: *Microsystem Technologies* 23.9 (2017), pp. 4203–4209. ISSN: 0946-7076. DOI: 10.1007/s00542-016-2842-2.

[43] Robert Puers. 'Capacitive sensors: When and how to use them'. In: *Sensors and Actuators A: Physical* 37-38 (1993), pp. 93–105. ISSN: 09244247. DOI: 10.1016/0924-4247(93)80019-D.

[44] S. Uejima et al. 'Fabrication of Miniaturized Capacitive Pressure Sensor using Thin Film Metallic Glass'. In: *MHS2018*. Ed. by Fumihito Arai and Jun Ota. [Piscataway, New Jersey]: IEEE, 2018, pp. 1–5. ISBN: 978-1-5386-6793-4. DOI: 10.1109/MHS.2018.8887020.

[45] Duy-Son Nguyen et al. 'MEMS-based capacitive pressure sensors with pre-stressed sensing diaphragms'. In: *IEEE SENSORS 2015*. Ed. by Hyung-Gi Byun. Piscataway, NJ: IEEE, 2015, pp. 1–4. ISBN: 978-1-4799-8203-5. DOI: 10.1109/ICSENS.2015.7370481.

[46] John Park and Steve Mackay. *Practical data acquisition for instrumentation and control systems*. Practical. Oxford, Burlington, MA: Newnes, 2003. ISBN: 9780750657969. DOI: 10.1016/B978-0-7506-5796-9.X5000-9.

[47] Joseph C. Doll and Beth L. Pruitt. *Piezoresistor design and applications*. Microsystems and nanosystems. New York: Springer, 2013. ISBN: 978-1-4614-8516-2. DOI: 10.1007/978-1-4614-8517-9.

[48] Byunghoon Bae et al. 'Design optimization of a piezoresistive pressure sensor considering the output signal-to-noise ratio'. In: *Journal of Micromechanics and Microengineering* 14.12 (2004), pp. 1597–1607. ISSN: 0960-1317. DOI: 10.1088/0960-1317/14/12/001.

[49] T. B. Gabrielson. 'Mechanical-thermal noise in micromachined acoustic and vibration sensors'. In: *IEEE Transactions on Electron Devices* 40.5 (1993), pp. 903–909. ISSN: 0018-9383. DOI: 10.1109/16.210197.

[50] R. R. Spender et al. 'A theoretical study of transducer noise in piezoresistive and capacitive silicon pressure sensors'. In: *IEEE Transactions on Electron Devices* 35.8 (1988), pp. 1289–1298. ISSN: 0018-9383. DOI: 10.1109/16.2550.

[51] Franco Maloberti. *Data converters*. Dordrecht: Springer, 2008. ISBN: 978-0-387-32485-2. DOI: 10.1007/978-0-387-32486-9.

[52] Walt Kester, ed. *Data conversion handbook*. Analog Devices series. Amsterdam and Heidelberg: Elsevier Newnes, 2007. ISBN: 9780750678414.

[53] *SM5420E Series Datasheet*. 2016. (Visited on 15/07/2020).

[54] J. Solis Arbustini et al. 'A 16-bits Pressure Sensing Interface Integrating a 460 fJ/conv Incremental Sigma Delta ADC for Medical Devices'. In: *LASCAS 2020 - 11th IEEE Latin American Symposium on Circuits and Systems*. 2020.

[55] Kofi A.A. Makinwa, Andrea Baschirotto and Pieter Harpe. *Efficient Sensor Interfaces, Advanced Amplifiers and Low Power RF Systems*. Cham: Springer International Publishing, 2016. ISBN: 978-3-319-21184-8. DOI: 10.1007/978-3-319-21185-5.

[56] José M. de La Rosa and Rocío del Río. *CMOS Sigma-Delta Converters: Practical design guide*. Chichester, West Sussex: Wiley IEEE Press, 2013. ISBN: 9781118569238. DOI: 10.1002/9781118569238.

[57] Alexander Mora Sánchez, Wolfgang Krautschneider and Holger Göbel. *Sigma-Delta analog-to-digital modulators with a single operational transconductance amplifier for low-power SoC design in biomedical applications: Zugl.:Hamburg-Harburg, Techn. Univ., Institut für Nanoelektronik, Diss., 2007*. Berichte aus der Elektronik. Aachen: Shaker, 2007. ISBN: 9783832267575.

[58] R. del Río et al. *CMOS Cascade Sigma-Delta Modulators for Sensors and Telecom: Error Analysis and Practical Design*. Analog Circuits and Signal Processing Series. Dordrecht: Springer, 2006. ISBN: 978-1-4020-4775-6. DOI: 10.1007/1-4020-4776-2.

[59] R. Jacob Baker. *CMOS: Circuit design, layout, and simulation*. Third edition. IEEE Press series on microelectronic systems. Hoboken, N.J: IEEE Press/Wiley, 2010. ISBN: 9780470891179. DOI: 10.1002/9780470891179.

[60] Yuming He et al. '27.7 A 0.05mm2 1V capacitance-to-digital converter based on period modulation'. In: *IEEE International Solid-State Circuits Conference (ISSCC), 2015*. Ed. by Laura Fujino. Piscataway, NJ: IEEE, 2015, pp. 1–3. ISBN: 978-1-4799-6223-5. DOI: 10.1109/ISSCC.2015.7063138.

[61] Sechang Oh et al. 'A Dual-Slope Capacitance-to-Digital Converter Integrated in an Implantable Pressure-Sensing System'. In: *IEEE Journal of Solid-State Circuits* 50.7 (2015), pp. 1581–1591. ISSN: 0018-9200. DOI: 10.1109/JSSC.2015.2435736.

[62] Sujin Park, Geon-Hwi Lee and SeongHwan Cho. 'A 2.69uW Dual Quantization-Based Capacitance-to-Digital Converter for Pressure, Humidity, and Acceleration Sensing in 0.18uWCMOS'. In: *2018 IEEE Symposium on VLSI Circuits*. IEEE, 6/18/2018 - 6/22/2018, pp. 163–164. ISBN: 978-1-5386-4214-6. DOI: 10.1109/VLSIC.2018.8502339.

[63] Ruimin Yang, Michiel A. P. Pertijs and Stoyan Nihtianov. 'A Precision Capacitance-to-Digital Converter With 16.7-bit ENOB and 7.5-ppm/°C Thermal Drift'. In: *IEEE Journal of Solid-State Circuits* 52.11 (2017), pp. 3018–3031. ISSN: 0018-9200. DOI: 10.1109/JSSC.2017.2734900.

[64] P. Mendoza Ponce et al. 'A Pressure Sensor with 0.30 mmHg Resolution incorporating a 4.19 pJ/conv Thyristor-based Capacitance-to-Time Converter for Intra-Corporeal Pressure Monitoring Applications'. In: *2019 IEEE Biomedical Circuits and Systems Conference (BioCAS)*. 2019, pp. 1–4. DOI: 10.1109/BIOCAS.2019.8919042.

[65] Timo Schary. 'Capacitive Surface-Micromachined Pressure Sensors on Fused Silica: Contributions to Micromachining on Fused Silica'. disertation. Germany: Universität Bremen, Jan, 2009.

[66] B. Chang, G. Kim and W. Kim. 'A Low Voltage Low Power CMOS Delay Element'. In: *ESSCIRC '95: Twenty-first European Solid-State Circuits Conference*. 1995, pp. 222–225.

[67] Gyudong Kim et al. 'A low-voltage, low-power CMOS delay element'. In: *IEEE Journal of Solid-State Circuits* 31.7 (1996), pp. 966–971. ISSN: 0018-9200. DOI: 10.1109/4.508210.

[68] John Paul Uyemura. *CMOS logic circuit design*. 4. printing. Boston: Kluwer Acad. Publ, 2003. ISBN: 9780792384526. DOI: 10.1007/b117409.

[69] Yu-Hsuan Chiang and Shen-Iuan Liu. 'A Submicrowatt 1.1-MHz CMOS Relaxation Oscillator With Temperature Compensation'. In: *IEEE Transactions on Circuits and Systems II: Express Briefs* 60.12 (2013), pp. 837–841. ISSN: 1549-7747. DOI: 10.1109/TCSII.2013.2281920.

[70] Deyan Levski, Martin Wany and Bhaskar Choubey. 'Ramp Noise Projection in CMOS Image Sensor Single-Slope ADCs'. In: *IEEE Transactions on Circuits and Systems I: Regular Papers* 64.6 (2017), pp. 1380–1389. ISSN: 1057-7122. DOI: 10.1109/TCSI.2017.2662950.

[71] A. A. Abidi. 'Phase Noise and Jitter in CMOS Ring Oscillators'. In: *IEEE Journal of Solid-State Circuits* 41.8 (2006), pp. 1803–1816. ISSN: 0018-9200. DOI: 10.1109/JSSC.2006.876206.

[72] Nicola Da Dalt and Ali Sheikholeslami. *Understanding jitter and phase noise: A circuits and systems perspective*. Cambridge: Cambridge University Press, 2018. ISBN: 9781107188570. DOI: 10.1017/9781316981238.

[73] Ali Grami. *Probability, random variables, statistics, and random processes: Fundamentals and applications*. Hoboken, NJ: John Wiley & Sons, 2020. ISBN: 1119300827.

[74] L. N. Alves and R. L. Aguiar. 'Noise performance of classical current mirrors'. In: *ICECS 2002*. Ed. by Adrijan Barić. Piscataway, NJ: IEEE Service Center, 2002, pp. 277–280. ISBN: 0-7803-7596-3. DOI: 10.1109/ICECS.2002.1045387.

[75] A. Hajimiri, S. Limotyrakis and T. H. Lee. 'Jitter and phase noise in ring oscillators'. In: *IEEE Journal of Solid-State Circuits* 34.6 (1999), pp. 790–804. ISSN: 0018-9200. DOI: 10.1109/4.766813.

[76] T. Sakurai and A. R. Newton. 'Alpha-power law MOSFET model and its applications to CMOS inverter delay and other formulas'. In: *IEEE Journal of Solid-State Circuits* 25.2 (1990), pp. 584–594. ISSN: 0018-9200. DOI: 10.1109/4.52187.

[77] S.L.J. Gierkink and E. van Tuij. 'A coupled sawtooth oscillator combining low jitter with high control linearity'. In: *IEEE Journal of Solid-State Circuits* 37.6 (2002), pp. 702–710. ISSN: 0018-9200. DOI: 10.1109/JSSC.2002.1004574.

[78] *Capacitive Pressure Sensors*. 2014. URL: http://www.protron-mikrotechnik.de/download/Protron-Pressure-Sensor-11_2014.pdf.

[79] Mihai A. T. Sanduleanu and A. J. M. Tuijl. *Power Trade-Offs and Low-Power in Analog CMOS ICs*. Vol. 662. The International Series in Engineering and Computer Science, Analog Circuits and Signal Processing. Boston, MA: Kluwer Academic Publishers, 2003. ISBN: 9780792376422. DOI: 10.1007/b100867. URL: http://site.ebrary.com/lib/academiccompletetitles/home.action.

[80] *Illustration of the pain pathway in René Descartes' Traite de l'homme (Treatise of Man) 1664*. URL: https://upload.wikimedia.org/wikipedia/commons/8/8a/Descartes-reflex.JPG (visited on 27/04/2020). In the public domain.

[81] B. J. Holtzclaw. 'Monitoring body temperature'. In: *AACN clinical issues in critical care nursing* 4.1 (1993), pp. 44–55. ISSN: 1046-7467.

[82] Zhiheng Zheng et al. 'A CMOS Temperature Sensor With Single-Point Calibration for Retinal Prosthesis'. In: *2018 IEEE Asia Pacific Conference on Circuits and Systems (APCCAS 2018)*. Piscataway, NJ: IEEE, 2018, pp. 147–150. ISBN: 978-1-5386-8240-1. DOI: 10.1109/APCCAS.2018.8605719.

[83] L. Michalski. *Temperature measurement*. 2nd ed. Chichester and New York: J. Wiley, 2001. ISBN: 9780471867791. DOI: 10.1002/0470846135.

[84] E. Velmre. 'Thomas Johann Seebeck and his contribution to the modern science and technology'. In: *12th Biennial Baltic Electronics Conference (BEC), 2010*. Piscataway, NJ: IEEE, 2010, pp. 17–24. ISBN: 978-1-4244-7356-4. DOI: 10.1109/BEC.2010.5631216.

[85] Ping Wang and Qingjun Liu. *Biomedical Sensors and Measurement*. Vol. 0. Advanced Topics in Science and Technology in China. Berlin, Heidelberg: Springer-Verlag Berlin Heidelberg, 2011. ISBN: 978-3-642-19524-2. DOI: 10.1007/978-3-642-19525-9.

[86] Michiel A.P. Pertijs and Johan H. Huijsing. *PRECISION TEMPERATURE SENSORS IN CMOS TECHNOLOGY*. Analog Circuits and Signal Processing. Dordrecht: Springer, 2006. ISBN: 978-1-4020-5257-6. DOI: 10.1007/1-4020-5258-8.

[87] Sining Pan et al. 'A Resistor-Based Temperature Sensor With a 0.13 pJ · K2 Resolution FoM'. In: *IEEE Journal of Solid-State Circuits* 53.1 (2018), pp. 164–173. ISSN: 0018-9200. DOI: 10.1109/JSSC.2017.2746671.

[88] Chen Zhao et al. 'A CMOS on-chip temperature sensor with −0.21°C 0.17 °C inaccuracy from −20 °C to 100 °C'. In: *IEEE International Symposium on Circuits and Systems (ISCAS), 2013*. Piscataway, NJ: IEEE, 2013, pp. 2621–2625. ISBN: 978-1-4673-5762-3. DOI: 10.1109/ISCAS.2013.6572416.

[89] Shuang Xie, Xiaoliang Ge and Albert Theuwissen. 'Temperature Sensors Incorporated into a CMOS Image Sensor with Column Zoom ADCs'. In: *2019 IEEE International Symposium on Circuits and Systems (ISCAS 2019)*. Piscataway, NJ: IEEE, 2019, pp. 1–5. ISBN: 978-1-7281-0397-6. DOI: 10.1109/ISCAS.2019.8702321.

[90] Pablo Ituero, Jose L. Ayala and Marisa Lopez-Vallejo. 'Leakage-based On-Chip Thermal Sensor for CMOS Technology'. In: *IEEE International Symposium on Circuits and Systems, 2007*. Piscataway, NJ: IEEE Service Center, 2007, pp. 3327–3330. ISBN: 1-4244-0920-9. DOI: 10.1109/ISCAS.2007.378223.

[91] G.C.M. Meijer, Guijie Wang and F. Fruett. 'Temperature sensors and voltage references implemented in CMOS technology'. In: *IEEE Sensors Journal* 1.3 (2001), pp. 225–234. ISSN: 1558-1748. DOI: 10.1109/JSEN.2001.954835.

[92] Ori Bass and Joseph Shor. 'A Miniaturized 0.003 mm^2 PNP-Based Thermal Sensor for Dense CPU Thermal Monitoring'. In: *IEEE Transactions on Circuits and Systems I: Regular Papers* (2020), pp. 1–9. ISSN: 1057-7122. DOI: 10.1109/TCSI.2020.2987595.

[93] Yan Lu and Chi-Seng Lam, eds. *Selected topics in power, RF, and mixed-signal ICs*. Tutorials in circuits and systems. Aalborg, Denmark: River Publishers, 2017. ISBN: 879360940X.

[94] Pieter Harpe, Kofi A. A. Makinwa and Andrea Baschirotto. *Hybrid ADCs, smart sensors for the IoT, and Sub-1V & advanced node analog circuit design: Advances in analog circuit design 2017*. Cham: Springer, 2018. ISBN: 978-3-319-61284-3. DOI: 10.1007/978-3-319-61285-0.

[95] Behzad Razavi. *Design of analog CMOS integrated circuits*. McGraw-Hill series in electrical and computer engineering. Boston Burr Ridge, IL et al.: McGraw-Hill, 2001. ISBN: 978-0072380323. URL: http://www.loc.gov/catdir/description/mh021/00044789.html.

[96] *Metronome from PSF Project*. URL: https://commons.wikimedia.org/wiki/File:Metronome_(PSF).png (visited on 27/04/2020). Public domain.

[97] Pablo Mendoza Ponce et al. 'A 1.9 nW Timer and Clock Generation Unit for Low Data-Rate Implantable Medical Devices'. In: *2020 IEEE 11th Latin American Symposium on Circuits & Systems (LASCAS)*. IEEE, 2/25/2020 - 2/28/2020, pp. 1–4. ISBN: 978-1-7281-3427-7. DOI: 10.1109/LASCAS45839.2020.9068949.

[98] Dominic A. Funke et al. 'Ultra low-power, -area and -frequency CMOS thyristor based oscillator for autonomous microsystems'. In: *2015 Nordic Circuits and Systems Conference (NORCAS) NORCHIP & International Symposium on System-on-Chip (SoC)*. Ed. by Jim Tørresen. Piscataway, NJ: IEEE, 2015, pp. 1–4. ISBN: 978-1-4673-6576-5. DOI: 10.1109/NORCHIP.2015.7364414.

[99] Alice Wang, Benton H. Calhoun and Anantha P. Chandrakasan. *Subthreshold Design for Ultra Low-Power Systems*. Series on Integrated Circuits and Systems. Boston, MA: Springer Science+Business Media LLC, 2007. ISBN: 978-0-387-33515-5. DOI: 10.1007/978-0-387-34501-7.

[100] *A drawing of a nuclear-powered heart pacemaker developed by the ARCO Nuclear Company for the U.S. Atomic Energy Commission. Circa 1973.* 2020-04-13. URL: https://upload.wikimedia.org/wikipedia/commons/9/9b/HD.17.068_%2811966272974%29.jpg (visited on 27/04/2020). In the public domain.

[101] Wen H. Ko. 'Early History and Challenges of Implantable Electronics'. In: *ACM journal on emerging technologies in computing systems* 8.2 (2012), p. 8. ISSN: 1550-4832. DOI: 10.1145/2180878.2180880.

[102] J. Paulo Davim. *The design and manufacture of medical devices*. Vol. 4. Woodhead Publishing reviews. Cambridge: Woodhead Publishing Ltd, 2012. ISBN: 978-1-907568-72-5. URL: http://search.ebscohost.com/login.aspx?direct=true&scope=site&db=nlebk&AN=671043.

[103] Wen H. Ko and Thomas M. Spear. 'Packaging Materials and Techniques for Implantable Instruments'. In: *IEEE Engineering in Medicine and Biology Magazine* 2.1 (1983), pp. 24–38. ISSN: 0739-5175. DOI: 10.1109/EMB-M.1983.5005879.

[104] Vinny R. Sastri. *Plastics in medical devices: Properties, requirements, and applications*. Plastics Design Library. PDL handbook series. Burlington, Mass: William Andrew, 2010. ISBN: 9780815520276. URL: http://site.ebrary.com/lib/alltitles/docDetail.action?docID=10391674.

[105] Roger Narayan. *Biomedical Materials*. Boston, MA: Springer-Verlag US, 2009. ISBN: 978-0-387-84871-6. DOI: 10.1007/978-0-387-84872-3.

[106] Buddy D. Ratner, ed. *Biomaterials science: An introduction to materials in medicine*. 3. ed. Amsterdam and Heidelberg: Elsevier, 2013. ISBN: 9780080877808. URL: http://site.ebrary.com/lib/alltitles/docDetail.action?docID=10627998.

[107] Buddy D. Ratner. 'The biocompatibility manifesto: biocompatibility for the twenty-first century'. In: *Journal of cardiovascular translational research* 4.5 (2011), pp. 523–527. DOI: 10.1007/s12265-011-9287-x.

[108] Omer Can Akgun et al. 'A Chip Integrity Monitor for Evaluating Long-term Encapsulation Performance Within Active Flexible Implants'. In: *BioCAS 2019*. Piscataway, NJ: IEEE, 2019, pp. 1–4. ISBN: 978-1-5090-0617-5. DOI: 10.1109/BIOCAS.2019.8919203.

[109] Albert Kim, Charles R. Powell and Babak Ziaie. 'An Universal packaging technique for low-drift implantable pressure sensors'. In: *Biomedical microdevices* 18.2 (2016), p. 32. DOI: 10.1007/s10544-016-0058-y.

[110] Adam P. Fraise, J.-Y. Maillard and Syed Sattar. *Russell, Hugo & Ayliffe's Principles and practice of disinfection, preservation, and sterilization*. 5th ed. Chichester, U.K: Wiley-Blackwell, 2013. ISBN: 9781299158573. DOI: 10.1002/9781118425831. URL: http://site.ebrary.com/lib/alltitles/docDetail.action?docID=10657797.

[111] Kayvon Modjarrad and Sina Ebnesajjad, eds. *Handbook of polymer applications in medicine and medical devices*. PDL handbook series. Oxford: Andrew Elsevier, 2014. ISBN: 978-0-323-22805-3.

[112] Andreas Inmann and Diana Hodgins. *Implantable sensor systems for medical applications*. Vol. number 52. Woodhead Publishing series in biomaterials. Cambridge, UK: Woodhead Publishing Limited, 2013. ISBN: 978-1-84569-987-1. URL: http://site.ebrary.com/lib/alltitles/docDetail.action?docID=10767137.

[113] E. S. W. Kong. *Nanomaterials, Polymers and Devices: Materials Functionalization and Device Fabrication*. Hoboken: Wiley, 2015. ISBN: 9781118867204. DOI: 10.1002/9781118867204.

[114] Jay Han-Chieh Chang et al. 'Reliable packaging for parylene-based flexible retinal implant'. In: *Transducers & Eurosensors XXVII*. Piscataway, NJ: IEEE, 2013, pp. 2612–2615. ISBN: 978-1-4673-5983-2. DOI: 10.1109/Transducers.2013.6627341.

[115] K. C. Aw et al. 'A transparent and flexible organic bistable memory device using parylene with embedded gold nanoparticles'. In: *Journal of Materials Science: Materials in Electronics* 24.8 (2013), pp. 3116–3125. ISSN: 0957-4522. DOI: 10.1007/s10854-013-1219-x.

[116] Dirk J. Broer and Arnoldus J. M. van den Broek. 'Additive method of manufacturing metal patterns on synthetic resin substrates. United States Patent: 4259435'. URL: http://patft.uspto.gov/netacgi/nph-Parser?Sect1=PTO1&Sect2=HITOFF&p=1&u=/netahtml/PTO/srchnum.html&r=1&f=G&l=50&d=PALL&s1=4259435.PN. (visited on 24/05/2020).

[117] *MED4-4420 Low consistency silicone elastomer: Datasheet*. 11-26-2018. URL: https://www.avantorsciences.com/assetsvc/asset/en_US/id/29019199/contents/en_us_tds_nusimed4-4420.pdf.

[118] James J. Licari. *Coating materials for electronic applications: Polymers, processes, reliability, testing*. Materials and Processes for Electronic Applications Ser. Norwich, NY: Noyes Publications/William Andrew Publ, 2010. ISBN: 9780815516477. URL: http://www.sciencedirect.com/science/book/9780815514923.

[119] Haleh Ardebili and Michael Pecht. *Encapsulation technologies for electronic applications*. Materials and processes for electronic applications series. Oxford: William Andrew, 2009. ISBN: 0815515766. URL: http://site.ebrary.com/lib/alltitles/docDetail.action?docID=10349826.

[120] *Materials Data Sheet: Photopolymer Resin for Form1+ and Form 2*. 2019. URL: https://archive-media.formlabs.com/upload/XL-DataSheet.pdf.

[121] *SF33 - RTV2 Silikon (Silikonkautschuk)*. 5-28-2020. URL: https://www.silikonfabrik.de/silikone/sf-silikon/sf33-rtv2-silikon-silikonkautschuk.html.

[122] *ACHEM - Produktinfo SG-1008*. 6-21-2018. URL: http://www.achem.de/SG-1008.html.

[123] Dominick V. Rosato, Donald V. Rosato and Marlene G. Rosato, eds. *Injection Molding Handbook*. Third Edition. Boston, MA and s.l.: Springer US, 2000. ISBN: 9781461370772. DOI: 10.1007/978-1-4615-4597-2.

[124] *MED1-161 Silicone primer: Datasheet*. 11-13-2018. URL: https://www.avantorsciences.com/assetsvc/asset/en_US/id/29018178/contents/en_us_tds_nusimed1-161.pdf.

[125] P. Mendoza Ponce et al. '3D-printing technology as a tool for medical implantable electronic devices'. In: *Transactions on Additive Manufacturing Meets Medicine* 1.1 (2019), pp. 21–22. DOI: 10.18416/AMMM.2019.1909S02T03.

[126] *Clear Photoreactive Resin for Form 1, Form 1+, Form 2 - Safety data sheet: [Material safety data Sheet]*. 2016. URL: https://archive-media.formlabs.com/upload/Clear-SDS_u324bsC.pdf.

[127] Juliane Kuhl et al. 'Additively manufactured anatomical heart model for performance evaluation of aortic valve implants: Transactions on Additive Manufacturing Meets Medicine, Vol 2 No 1 (2020): Trans. AMMM / Transactions on Additive Manufacturing Meets Medicine, Vol 2 No 1 (2020): Trans. AMMM'. In: (2020). DOI: 10.18416/AMMM.2020.2009027.

[128] *Clara Jacobi*. 2020-05-04. URL: http://resource.nlm.nih.gov/101392944 (visited on 04/05/2020). In the public domain.

[129] James Stuart Olson. *The history of cancer: An annotated bibliography*. Vol. 3. Bibliographies and indexes in medical studies. New York, N.Y.: Greenwood Press, 1989. ISBN: 0313258899.

[130] Stewart W. B, Wild P. C and International Agency for Research on Cancer. *World Cancer Report 2014*. Geneva: IARC, 2014. ISBN: 9789283204343.

[131] G. Kroemer et al. *Oncogenes Meet Metabolism: From Deregulated Genes to a Broader Understanding of Tumour Physiology*. 1. Aufl. Vol. 2007/4. Ernst Schering Research Foundation Workshop. s.l.: Springer-Verlag, 2008. ISBN: 978-3-540-79477-6. DOI: 10.1007/978-3-540-79478-3.

[132] Alexander Birbrair. *Tumor microenvironment: Recent advances*. Vol. v. 1225. Advances in Experimental Medicine and Biology. Cham: Springer, 2020. ISBN: 978-3-030-35726-9. DOI: 10.1007/978-3-030-35727-6.

[133] Dietmar W. Siemann. *Tumor microenvironment*. Chichester, West Sussex: Wiley, 2011. ISBN: 9780470669891. DOI: 10.1002/9780470669891.

[134] Chandra P. Sharma, ed. *Biointegration of medical implant materials*. Second edition. Woodhead Publishing series in biomaterials. Duxford: Woodhead Publishing, an imprint of Elsevier, 2020. ISBN: 978-0-08-102680-9.

[135] Gulcen Yeldag, Alistair Rice and Armando Del Río Hernández. 'Chemoresistance and the Self-Maintaining Tumor Microenvironment'. In: *Cancers* 10.12 (2018). ISSN: 2072-6694. DOI: 10.3390/cancers10120471.

[136] Yu Yu and Jiuwei Cui. 'Present and future of cancer immunotherapy: A tumor microenvironmental perspective'. In: *Oncology letters* 16.4 (2018), pp. 4105–4113. ISSN: 1792-1074. DOI: 10.3892/ol.2018.9219.

[137] Christian R. Gomez. *Tumor Hypoxia: Impact in Tumorigenesis, Diagnosis, Prognosis and Therapeutics*. s.l.: Frontiers Media SA, 2017. ISBN: 9782889450640. URL: http://www.doabooks.org/doab?func=fulltext&rid=22916.

[138] Jacinta Serpa. *Tumor Microenvironment: The Main Driver of Metabolic Adaptation*. Vol. 1219. Advances in Experimental Medicine and Biology Ser. New York and Berlin: Springer and Springer [Distributor], March 2020. ISBN: 978-3-030-34024-7. DOI: 10.1007/978-3-030-34025-4.

[139] Domenico Ribatti. *History of Research on Tumor Angiogenesis*. Dordrecht: Springer Netherlands, 2009. ISBN: 978-1-4020-9559-7. DOI: 10.1007/978-1-4020-9563-4.

[140] Agnieszka Zimna and Maciej Kurpisz. 'Hypoxia-Inducible Factor-1 in Physiological and Pathophysiological Angiogenesis: Applications and Therapies'. In: *BioMed research international* 2015 (2015), p. 549412. DOI: 10.1155/2015/549412.

[141] Valgerdur G. Halldorsdottir et al. 'Subharmonic-Aided Pressure Estimation for Monitoring Interstitial Fluid Pressure in Tumors: Calibration and Treatment with Paclitaxel in Breast Cancer Xenografts'. In: *Ultrasound in medicine & biology* 43.7 (2017), pp. 1401–1410. DOI: 10.1016/j.ultrasmedbio.2017.02.011.

[142] Shawn Stapleton et al. 'Radiation and Heat Improve the Delivery and Efficacy of Nanotherapeutics by Modulating Intratumoral Fluid Dynamics'. In: *ACS nano* 12.8 (2018), pp. 7583–7600. DOI: 10.1021/acsnano.7b06301.

[143] Arindam Sen et al. 'Mild elevation of body temperature reduces tumor interstitial fluid pressure and hypoxia and enhances efficacy of radiotherapy in murine tumor models'. In: *Cancer research* 71.11 (2011), pp. 3872–3880. DOI: 10.1158/0008-5472.CAN-10-4482.

[144] Catarina Roma-Rodrigues et al. 'Targeting Tumor Microenvironment for Cancer Therapy'. In: *International journal of molecular sciences* 20.4 (2019). DOI: 10.3390/ijms20040840.

[145] Elizabeth A. Repasky, Sharon S. Evans and Mark W. Dewhirst. 'Temperature matters! And why it should matter to tumor immunologists'. In: *Cancer immunology research* 1.4 (2013), pp. 210–216. DOI: 10.1158/2326-6066.CIR-13-0118.

[146] Seung Hyun Song et al. 'An Implantable Wireless Interstitial Pressure Sensor With Integrated Guyton Chamber: in vivo Study in Solid Tumors'. In: *IEEE transactions on bio-medical engineering* 63.11 (2016), pp. 2273–2277. DOI: 10.1109/TBME.2016.2522460.

[147] Qianyun Zhang et al. 'Effect of Ultrasound Combined With Microbubble Therapy on Interstitial Fluid Pressure and VX2 Tumor Structure in Rabbit'. In: *Frontiers in pharmacology* 10 (2019), p. 716. ISSN: 1663-9812. DOI: 10.3389/fphar.2019.00716.

[148] A. C. Guyton. 'A concept of negative interstitial pressure based on pressures in implanted perforated capsules'. In: *Circulation research* 12 (1963), pp. 399–414. ISSN: 0009-7330. DOI: 10.1161/01.res.12.4.399.

[149] P. F. Scholander, A. R. Hargens and S. L. Miller. 'Negative pressure in the interstitial fluid of animals. Fluid tensions are spectacular in plants; in animals they are elusively small, but just as vital'. In: *Science (New York, N.Y.)* 161.3839 (1968), pp. 321–328. ISSN: 0036-8075. DOI: 10.1126/science.161.3839.321.

[150] H. O. Fadnes, R. K. Reed and K. Aukland. 'Interstitial fluid pressure in rats measured with a modified wick technique'. In: *Microvascular Research* 14.1 (1977), pp. 27–36. ISSN: 00262862. DOI: 10.1016/0026-2862(77)90138-8.

[151] Eve LoCastro et al. 'Computational Modeling of Interstitial Fluid Pressure and Velocity in Head and Neck Cancer Based on Dynamic Contrast-Enhanced Magnetic Resonance Imaging: Feasibility Analysis'. In: *Tomography (Ann Arbor, Mich.)* 6.2 (2020), pp. 129–138. DOI: 10.18383/j.tom.2020.00005.

[152] H. Wiig, R. K. Reed and K. Aukland. 'Measurement of interstitial fluid pressure: comparison of methods'. In: *Annals of Biomedical Engineering* 14.2 (1986), pp. 139–151. ISSN: 1573-9686. DOI: 10.1007/BF02584264.

[153] Simon Walker-Samuel et al. 'Investigating Low-Velocity Fluid Flow in Tumors with Convection-MRI'. In: *Cancer research* 78.7 (2018), pp. 1859–1872. DOI: 10.1158/0008-5472.CAN-17-1546.

[154] Rasha Elmghirbi et al. 'Toward a noninvasive estimate of interstitial fluid pressure by dynamic contrast-enhanced MRI in a rat model of cerebral tumor'. In: *Magnetic resonance in medicine* 80.5 (2018), pp. 2040–2052. DOI: 10.1002/mrm.27163.

[155] J. F. Head et al. 'The important role of infrared imaging in breast cancer'. In: *IEEE Engineering in Medicine and Biology Magazine* 19.3 (2000), pp. 52–57. ISSN: 0739-5175. DOI: 10.1109/51.844380.

[156] Sumita Mishra et al. 'Breast Cancer Detection using Thermal Images and Deep Learning'. In: *2020 7th International Conference on Computing for Sustainable Global Development (INDIACom)*, pp. 211–216. DOI: 10.23919/INDIACom49435.2020.9083722.

[157] Chengli Song et al. 'Thermographic assessment of tumor growth in mouse xenografts'. In: *International Journal of Cancer* 121.5 (2007), pp. 1055–1058. ISSN: 00207136. DOI: 10.1002/ijc.22808.

[158] Qi Zhao et al. 'Use of a thermocouple for malignant tumor detection. Investigating temperature difference as a diagnostic criterion'. In: *IEEE Engineering in Medicine and Biology Magazine* 27.1 (2008), pp. 64–66. ISSN: 0739-5175. DOI: 10.1109/MEMB.2007.913292.

[159] Wei Xie et al. 'Evaluation of the ability of digital infrared imaging to detect vascular changes in experimental animal tumours'. In: *International Journal of Cancer* 108.5 (2004), pp. 790–794. ISSN: 00207136. DOI: 10.1002/ijc.11618.

[160] P. Mendoza Ponce, D. Schroeder and W. H. Krautschneider. 'Tradeoff Study on Switched Capacitor Regulators for Implantable Medical Devices'. In: *ICTOpen 2017 Conference Proceedings*. 2017, pp. 4–7.

[161] P. Mendoza Ponce et al. 'Super-capacitors for implantable medical devices with wireless power transmission'. In: *2018 14th Conference on Ph.D. Research in Microelectronics and Electronics (PRIME)*. 2018, pp. 241–244. DOI: 10.1109/PRIME.2018.8430360.

[162] Pierre Squara, Michael Imhoff and Maurizio Cecconi. 'Metrology in medicine: from measurements to decision, with specific reference to anesthesia and intensive care'. In: *Anesthesia and analgesia* 120.1 (2015), pp. 66–75. DOI: 10.1213/ANE.0000000000000477.

[163] Alan S. Morris. *Measurement and instrumentation principles*. Reprinted. Amsterdam: Elsevier Butterworth Heinemann, 2006. ISBN: 9780750650816. DOI: 10.1016/B978-0-7506-5081-6.X5000-0.

[164] M.M.B. Amer. 'Optimal design of experiment for medical sensors calibration'. In: *2001 conference proceedings of the 23rd Annual International Conference of the IEEE Engineering in Medicine and Biology Society, 25-28 October 2001, Istanbul, Turkey*. Ed. by Yorgo Istefanopulos. Piscataway, NJ: IEEE/EMB, 2001, pp. 3090–3095. ISBN: 0-7803-7211-5. DOI: 10.1109/IEMBS.2001.1017455.

[165] *CFR - Code of Federal Regulations Title 21*. 18.06.2020. URL: https://www.accessdata.fda.gov/scripts/cdrh/cfdocs/cfcfr/CFRSearch.cfm?fr=820.72.

[166] Janusz Bryzek. 'Introduction to IEEE-P1451, the emerging hardware-independent communication standard for smart transducers'. In: *Sensors and Actuators A: Physical* 62.1-3 (1997), pp. 711–723. ISSN: 09244247. DOI: 10.1016/S0924-4247(97)01536-7.

[167] Guanwu Zhou et al. 'A smart high accuracy silicon piezoresistive pressure sensor temperature compensation system'. In: *Sensors (Basel, Switzerland)* 14.7 (2014), pp. 12174–12190. DOI: 10.3390/s140712174.

[168] David Dagan Feng. *Biomedical Information Technology*. 2nd ed. Academic Press, 2020. ISBN: 978-0-12-816034-3.

[169] Jacob Fraden. *Handbook of Modern Sensors: Physics, Designs, and Applications*. 5th ed. 2016. Cham and New York: Springer, 2016. ISBN: 978-3-319-19302-1. DOI: 10.1007/978-3-319-19303-8.

[170] H. J. Oguey and D. Aebischer. 'CMOS current reference without resistance'. In: *IEEE Journal of Solid-State Circuits* 32.7 (1997), pp. 1132–1135. ISSN: 0018-9200. DOI: 10.1109/4.597305.

[171] G. Sayed et al. 'Ultra-Low-Power Self-Biased 1 nA Current Reference Circuit for Medical Monitoring Devices in 350 nm and 180 nm CMOS Technology'. In: *ANALOG 2018; 16th GMM/ITG-Symposium*, pp. 1–4.

Lebenslauf

Personal information

Last Name:	Mendoza Ponce
First Name:	Pablo
Nationality:	Costa Rican
Birth date:	29.11.1985
Birth place:	San José, Costa Rica

Studies

02/2003-02/2009	**Licentiate degree** in **Electronics Engineering**, Tecnológico de Costa Rica (TEC), San José, Costa Rica
10/2010-12/2012	**Master of Science** in **Telecommunications Engineering**, thesis on **Reconfigurable Software-Defined Receiver Algorithms for OFDM Systems**, Politecnico di Torino (POLITO), Turin, Italy
10/2015-08/2021	**Doctoral Studies** on **Implantable Medical Systems for the Invasive Monitoring of Pressure and Temperature** at the Institute for Integrated Circuits, Hamburg University of Technology (TUHH), Hamburg, Germany

Working experience

06/2009-03/2010	**Engineer** at the Research and Development Department, Canam Technologies inc., Cartago, Costa Rica
07/2013-09/2015	**Engineer** at the Hewlett-Packard Networking Research and Development Division, Softtek Costa Rica (outsourcing), Heredia, Costa Rica
07/2013-09/2015	**Lecturer** at the Electronics Engineering Program, Tecnológico de Costa Rica (TEC), Cartago, Costa Rica

07/2013-09/2015	**Lecturer** at the Computer Science Engineering Program Tecnológico de Costa Rica (TEC), Cartago, Costa Rica
10/2015-01/2021	**Research Assistant** at the Institute for Integrated Circuits Hamburg University of Technology (TUHH), Hamburg, Germany
07/2013-Present	**Lecturer** at the Electronics Engineering Department, Tecnológico de Costa Rica (TEC), San José, Costa Rica

List of Publications

[1] Juliane Kuhl, Pablo Daniel Mendoza Ponce, Wolfgang Krautschneider and Dieter Krause. 'Additively manufactured anatomical heart model for performance evaluation of aortic valve implants: Transactions on Additive Manufacturing Meets Medicine, Vol 2 No 1 (2020): Trans. AMMM / Transactions on Additive Manufacturing Meets Medicine, Vol 2 No 1 (2020): Trans. AMMM'. In: (2020). DOI: 10.18416/AMMM.2020.2009027.

[2] Pablo Mendoza Ponce, Gayas Sayed, Lait Abu Saleh, Wolfgang H. Krautschneider and Matthias Kuhl. 'A 1.9 nW Timer and Clock Generation Unit for Low Data-Rate Implantable Medical Devices'. In: *2020 IEEE 11th Latin American Symposium on Circuits & Systems (LASCAS)*. IEEE, 2/25/2020 - 2/28/2020, pp. 1–4. ISBN: 978-1-7281-3427-7. DOI: 10.1109/LASCAS45839.2020.9068949.

[3] Johan Solis-Arbustini, Pablo Mendoza-Ponce, Wolfgang H. Krautschneider and Matthias Kuhl. 'A 16-bit Pressure Sensing Interface Integrating a 460 fJ/conv Incremental Sigma Delta ADC for Medical Devices'. In: *2020 IEEE 11th Latin American Symposium on Circuits & Systems (LASCAS)*. IEEE, 2/25/2020 - 2/28/2020, pp. 1–4. ISBN: 978-1-7281-3427-7. DOI: 10.1109/LASCAS45839.2020.9068978.

[4] P. Mendoza Ponce, G. Sayed, L. Abu Saleh, W. H. Krautschneider and M. Kuhl. 'A Pressure Sensor with 0.30 mmHg Resolution incorporating a 4.19 pJ/conv Thyristor-based Capacitance-to-Time Converter for Intra-Corporeal Pressure Monitoring Applications'. In: *2019 IEEE Biomedical Circuits and Systems Conference (BioCAS)*. 2019, pp. 1–4. DOI: 10.1109/BIOCAS.2019.8919042.

[5] P. Mendoza Ponce, L. Abu Saleh, W. H. Krautschneider and M. Kuhl. '3D-printing technology as a tool for medical implantable electronic devices'. In: *Transactions on Additive Manufacturing Meets Medicine* 1.1 (2019), pp. 21–22. DOI: 10.18416/AMMM.2019.1909S02T03.

[6] G. Sayed, P. Mendoza Ponce, W. Krautschneider and M. Kuhl. 'Ultra-Low-Power Self-Biased 1 nA Current Reference Circuit for Medical Monitoring Devices in 350 nm and 180 nm CMOS Technology'. In: *ANALOG 2018; 16th GMM/ITG-Symposium*, pp. 1–4.

[7] P. Mendoza Ponce, B. John, D. Schroeder and W. H. Krautschneider. 'Super-capacitors for implantable medical devices with wireless power transmission'. In: *2018 14th Conference on Ph.D. Research in Microelectronics and Electronics (PRIME)*. 2018, pp. 241–244. DOI: 10.1109/PRIME.2018.8430360.

[8] P. Mendoza Ponce, D. Schroeder and W. H. Krautschneider. 'Trade-off Study on Switched Capacitor Regulators for Implantable Medical Devices'. In: *ICTOpen 2017 Conference Proceedings*. 2017, pp. 4–7.

[9] R. Ranjan, M. Hansen, P. Mendoza Ponce, L. Abu Saleh, D. Schroeder, M. Ziegler, H. Kohlstedt and W. H. Krautschneider. 'Integration of Double Barrier Memristor Die with Neuron ASIC for Neuromorphic Hardware Learning'. In: *2018 IEEE International Symposium on Circuits and Systems (ISCAS)*. 2018, pp. 1–5. DOI: 10.1109/ISCAS.2018.8350996.

[10] R. Ranjan, P. Mendoza Ponce, Wolf Lukas Hellweg, Alexandros Kyrmanidis, L. Abu Saleh, D. Schroeder and W. H. Krautschneider. 'Integrated Circuit with Memristor Emulator Array and Neuron Circuits for Biologically Inspired Neuromorphic Pattern Recognition'. In: *Journal of Circuits, Systems and Computers* 26.11 (2017), p. 1750183. ISSN: 0218-1266. DOI: 10.1142/S0218126617501833.

[11] R. Ranjan, A. Kyrmanidis, W. L. Hellweg, P. Mendoza Ponce, L. Abu Saleh, D. Schroeder and W. H. Krautschneider. 'Integrated circuit with memristor emulator array and neuron circuits for neuromorphic pattern recognition'. In: *2016 39th International Conference on Telecommunications and Signal Processing (TSP)*. 2016, pp. 265–268. DOI: 10.1109/TSP.2016.7760875.

[12] R. Ranjan, P. Mendoza Ponce, A. Kankuppe, B. John, L. Abu Saleh, D. Schroeder and W. H. Krautschneider. 'Programmable memristor emulator ASIC for biologically inspired memristive learning'. In: *2016 39th International Conference on Telecommunications and Signal Processing (TSP)*. 2016, pp. 261–264. DOI: 10.1109/TSP.2016.7760874.